TAKING CONTROL
COMPASSIONATELY

*Stories of the unique human spirit
inherent in Multiple Sclerosis nurses globally*

By Jillian Kingsford Smith

Taking Control Compassiontely: Stories of the unique human spirit inherent in Multiple Sclerosis nurses globally.

ISBN: 9780987537546 (paperback)
Copyright © 2020 Jillian Kingsford Smith
1st published 2020 by Take20 Stories, Brisbane Qld Australia
www.take20stories.com

Liability Disclaimer: The material contained in this book is general in nature and does not represent professional advice. It is not intended to provide specific guidance for particular circumstances and it should not be relied on as a basis for any decisions to take action on any matter that it covers. Readers should obtain professional or medical advice before acting on any information in this book. Neither the Author nor the Publisher can be held responsible for any loss or claim arising out of the use, or misuse, of the suggestions made or the failure to take medical advice.

National Library of Australia Cataloguing-in-publication data:

NATIONAL LIBRARY OF AUSTRALIA

A catalogue record for this work is available from the National Library of Australia

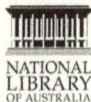

Cover Design: Vanessa Maynard.

DEDICATION

To my own MS Nurse,

Kaye Hooper

"I'm never afraid with you."
- Winnie the Pooh

ALSO BY JILLIAN KINGSFORD SMITH

Taking Control
A collection of inspiring stories for people living with MS

....

Taking Control Together

Real life stories on caring for yourself and a loved one with MS

....

Visit **www.take20stories.com** for more information.

CONTENTS

FOREWORD

*She took these stories and experiences and she wove them around
her own special understandings...*

....

Jillian Kingsford Smith. Connected to this name is the most
genuine example of humanness and service to others that you
can imagine. Sure, she is a writer, a journalist and very good with
words. But, most importantly, Jillian is someone who has given
so much of her own time to tell the stories of others, for others.
No agenda, no hidden messages, no other reasons. Just to leave a
mark and increase the visibility and awareness of MS as a disease and
as a life condition. An angel in human form, although she would
never see herself in this way.

You see, Jillian would never tell you this herself, but she had a
pretty rocky and inhumane entry into the world of being a patient.
Imagine battling through a self-described 'messy' marital separation
and all that entails - in moving houses and financial stress - when
Jillian started having weird symptoms that she had absolutely no
time nor inclination for. Ending up in the ER on a Friday night is
horrendous at the best of times, but it marked the start of a
whirlwind of possible diagnoses, stroke and MS at the forefront.
How could this be happening? "Be strong" became her mantra as
she then negotiated the confirmation of the diagnosis of MS and

how to tell that story to her loving family and many friends, one she didn't understand herself. Getting through that time was sheer hell on wheels. And then ten weeks later, a double whammy. The terror of finding a breast lump turned into a nightmare as breast cancer was confirmed and a mad rush into surgery, followed by chemotherapy and radiotherapy. You have got to be joking me. Seriously? This was Jillian's introduction into the world of being a patient. How could anyone bear this much? And bear it she did, and then some. And then some more. Yes, Jillian chose the much higher road.

Let me tell you about how Jillian came together. One of the stories you will read in this book is about one of Australia's foremost and respected MS Nurses, Kaye Hooper (Cameron). Well, Kaye is something of a celebrity in MS nursing in Australia, she has been around since the inception of MS nursing in this country and has been at the forefront of developing a network of MS Nurses in Australasia. Kaye was instrumental in bringing Jillian and I together. Kaye was Jillian's MS Nurse in Brisbane and a very important part of Jillian's life. And mine too as my mentor and confidante on all things MS and nursing. Kaye brought us together in the very embryonic stages of this book when it was just an idea to see if I could help Jillian connect with international nurses who might be willing to tell their story. It was the start of a beautiful friendship that mirrored my journey writing my PhD thesis, and Jillian's starting to get this book together. Jillian's work helped me develop my writing skills and I helped Jillian make the connections she needed to see if this book could indeed become a reality. We became a little team and each other's number one cheerleader. I was telling patient stories that reflected what Jillian was going through, and Jillian was telling MS Nurse stories that mirrored what I was going through. In a way, we were sort of running a parallel race, but one we couldn't see at the time, nor one that we ever formally identified. Until now. It is remarkably clear.

During my time as a MS Nurse, I served as a Board Member for the Multiple Sclerosis International Certification Board for many years. This was the platform where I met so many of my colleagues from all around the world, the MS Nurses from countries I had never been to, but we were sharing our lives and we all had a passion for our fellow MS Nurses in education and support, as well as our patients. Some of the most incredible souls I have ever met, and many of their stories are included here for you to enjoy, to learn from and to better understand the challenges and highlights of working not just in healthcare, but in MS in particular.

So, two peas in a pod, we started discussing so many things that started to resonate with us both. The idea for this book, purely Jillian's as part of her planned trilogy following on from stories of people living with MS in her first book, and then carers who love people living with MS in her second book, was fast becoming a reality. I connected Jillian with the many brilliant and selfless MS Nurses I have been fortunate to meet all around the globe so that Jillian could get a truly international perspective on life as a MS Nurse. The similarities, the subtle differences, the enormous differences, the individual stories. I trusted my colleagues with Jillian because I knew that she would look after them and coax the stories in a sensitive and thoughtful way, not just looking for a grab or a headline, but truly understanding where a person has come from and what makes them the unique person they are. I also knew I was going to probably learn so much more about these colleagues through Jillian and her distinctive lens, and many things I would never have ever guessed or ever known about. It was an exciting time for Jillian as she forged many new friendships with MS Nurses during the interview process. On many occasions I was contacted by the MS Nurses afterwards to tell me what a cathartic and wonderful experience it was and how respectful and sensitive Jillian was. I was so proud and happy that Jillian's dream was also benefitting so many MS Nurses and allowing them to let their stories soar.

Nursing in the world of MS is bloody hard. Some days are diamonds and some days are absolute stinkers. Thankfully, most days are somewhere in the middle! In such a unique role, MS Nurses are mostly at the forefront of the patient experience and essentially live and breathe their patients and all of the challenges, heartache, joys and decisions with them. To truly capture this in a way that others can understand, well, it probably hasn't been done on this scale before because it sort of sounds, well, impossible. But Jillian knew what to do. She took these stories and experiences and she wove them around her own special understandings to tell each MS Nurse's story in a way that both honours them and speaks the truth. My own story reflected things back to me I did not want to see, things I asked Jillian to remove because I did not want anyone to think badly of me if they knew about the secret, 'bad' stuff. The things that took my 'always there in public' smile away. The things that darkened my heart. But, Jillian convinced me that these things are what makes the story, the things people needed to know to understand what we go through, what makes us tick and what it is like for our loved ones supporting us at home so we can be there for others. So, they stayed in. For me, and for many others.

Readers, what do I hope you take away from Jillian's final book in this trilogy that can help you understand the world of MS a little better? Firstly, for people living with MS, loving someone living with MS or working alongside someone living with MS, welcome to the real MS world! Jillian's previous books have always reminded us what it feels like for those people, what they go through, often in secret or invisible to others. Now, this book tells the story of those caring for all of you and what is invisible to you most of the time, if not all of the time. The vulnerabilities, the hardships, the difficult days. But also, the highlights, the wonderful moments, the love that we have as MS Nurses for our job and for our patients. I know these days in nursing there has been a trend to keep it all professional and address people as clients, and us as health professionals, but

I don't believe any of that. There is love and respect between MS Nurses and their patients. We talk about the most intimate, difficult and special things together. We go beyond boundaries and beyond invisible lines. And now you get to see what it's really like. In the trenches providing a view of the MS world you have very likely never seen before. Secondly, I hope that you take away the hope that MS Nurses invest in every day and the very special role they have in MS care. And the depth and breadth of that feeling, because I happen to think it is an amazing and incredible phenomenon that marks MS Nurses as truly special. As Jillian reminded us in her second book 'Taking Control Together,' from the words of A.A Milne: "Some people care too much. I think it's called love." Never truer.

Finally, I want to thank Jillian on behalf of all the MS Nurses interviewed in the development of this book, and on behalf of all the MS Nurses who will be better understood by their patients as a result of these stories from Jillian. As I mentioned at the beginning, to comprehend that someone has spent more than three years totally devoted to a project and the huge amount of physical, emotional and mental effort this has taken, all to benefit others and not themselves, is a little hard to process. Yet Jillian has done this for us, as MS Nurses, to increase awareness about our role and to bring attention to the crucial role we play in many lives, sometimes the forgotten piece of the puzzle in a busy MS care circle. Jillian, we thank you and owe you so much. Thank you for bringing light into our world, just as you bring light into ours with your passion and insight. We are truly indebted.

Therese Burke RN MSCN PhD
Sydney, Australia
December 2019

INTRODUCTION

"Is there a burden in feeling like you can't have a bad day?
Absolutely. The hand-wringing irony is that we give our patients
the permission to have a bad day; to scream and shout and get
the emotion out so as they can find a release and bounce back.
But I just can't. On those days when I would go into the clinic
and my head just wasn't really in the space, or when I was feeling
a bit off because there's other things going on in life,
I could never allow myself to show a bad day."

- Therese Burke

A specialist nurse is one of the first people you will meet and speak to after you have been told you have a life-changing illness. They sit beside you as you try to get your mind around the quagmire of chaos you have just found yourself dumped in. Indeed, they will hold your hand and help you process the diagnosis and then gently guide you through those scary and uncertain early days.

Medicine – nor advice – can be given in a vacuum and it's often the nurse's role to figure out what else is going on in their patient's life so they can best support them.

And in that way, specialist nurses become a one stop shop. As the stories throughout this book will illustrate, they can be considered part psychologist, part councillor, part clinician, part medical interpreter, part social worker, part educator, part mediator…. and the list goes on.

The most common question that MS nurses will be asked after someone has been told "you have MS" is "are you sure?" followed very quickly by "what do I do now?"

"For a lot of patients, the biggest support we can provide is to simply re-assure that help is at hand; that I am on the end of a phone line; that they are not alone. And sometimes I can't solve any definitive problems, but I can at least listen to them or let them know if something sounds 'normal' and isn't worth worrying about. I have a lot of conversations that start off with people saying "Kaye, this might sound a bit strange but…" But nothing sounds strange any longer; I have heard it all!

"But really and truly it's all too much to take in right after you've been told you have multiple sclerosis. I prefer to explain that I'm going to take the person on a trip a bit like a 'highlights of Europe' trip that takes 21 days. We're going to see a little bit of everything, but you have to know that you'll want to come back and visit the stuff that really interests you later on."

- Kaye Hooper

Specialist nurses often live with the condition they're treating via proxy. Time and again as I was interviewing the nurses and writing their stories, I was overwhelmed by the similarity between how my subjects deal with MS and the emotional rollercoaster they ride with us. The emotional divide between patient and nurse is not as great as either would think. We experience the highs and lows of an unpredictable disease together. Just as many patients have inspired their nurses by their strength and courage, so too are the patients inspired and empowered by the guidance and compassion that their nurses show them.

There are recent studies that explore how the strength of the nurse/ patient relationship effects the treatment process and indeed the quality of life in the chronically ill. Across all the studies it was clear that a meaningful connection between the nurse and patient greatly influences the patient in wanting to achieve a positive outlook and successful outcome of the treatment.

Stories are a fundamental dimension of human experience, and nursing practice and story theory describes a narrative that occurs through intentional nurse-to-patient dialogue. From a nursing stance, careful attention is paid to the patient's story because it would lead to the essence of the person they're treating.

Throughout the two years of researching and interviewing for Taking Control Compassionately, it became obvious that the stories of these nurses are as much for people living with a chronic illness as they are for people considering a career as a specialist nurse. In fact, the two audiences became impossible to separate, so intricately intertwined were their psyche.

And the stories in this book provide a 360-degree view of specialist nursing and particularly in treating MS through discussing topics such as:

• The universal creativity required in nursing and the necessity of this creativity to support the patient.

• The importance of story theory in nursing.

• The ritual of medicine and how some traditions and practices set the scene for compassionate and successful nurse/patient relationships.

• The mental health challenges (and triumphs!) that both nurses and patients alike experience.

- The wide spectrum of patients treated by specialist nurses, from refugee and homeless populations right through to the complexity of paediatric patients. MS certainly doesn't discriminate and consequently the patient cohorts around the globe throw up many and varied experiences.

- The difficulties in treating and providing continuing care for patients in rural or remote locations.

- The inherent hope in research for the future treatment of MS, and in particular, the desire to see advances in personalised medicine for the targeted treatment of patient symptoms and disease course.

- The history of nursing, including the foundation of the most significant specialist nursing organisations around the globe and the development of landmark studies that would shape the treatment of MS.

- The formation of MS clinics internationally – from Beirut to Birmingham to Brisbane – and the cultural differences experienced in treating MS.

- Explanations of the development and evolution of the various diagnostic techniques for MS.

Most importantly, it is the personal accounts and excruciatingly honest anecdotes of these nurses that highlight the hidden and often enormous lengths MS nurses go to in providing care – and indeed better lives – for those they treat. These stories will guide patients with MS and their families as to how to live well with MS, but also provide comfort through illustrating the commonality of some of the challenges faced.

Similarly, the nurse's stories will provide deep insights for other nurses; ones that they can adapt and adopt within their own practice of patient management and self-care.

"This is a vocation that will absolutely shape you and that process for growth and learning is very important for nurses. Being able to spend time with patients provides a lasting imprint on your personality and psyche for ever. I've had patients who have left a lasting impression on my life and these experiences help us to help the next person."

- Joelle Massouh

I started developing this book series about six weeks after my own diagnosis of MS. I couldn't find any material that gave me the necessary information to form 'The Action Plan.' I didn't want to join a support group. In fact, I really didn't want to tell anyone at all that I was living with MS. If people knew I had MS they might think I was less capable... I'm not sure how I thought I was going to write a book about MS without telling anyone, but these are the small details we discard when we're on a mission!

Fast forward to eight years later and I can't deny I'm in disbelief that I've pulled off my dream of creating a 3-book series that looks at MS from every angle. The first book, 'Taking Control' became a best-seller and that brought the attention I was trying to avoid. Yep... the cat was definitely out of the bag. But oh my... the opportunities it has presented! MS Research Australia asked me to become one of their first ambassadors for the Kiss Goodbye to MS campaign, which a few short years later went global, I have spoken at Australia's Parliament House on World MS Day – as well as many an event to build awareness around living well with MS – and I've been invited to work with some incredibly bright and inspiring people along the way in the fields of advocacy, philanthropy, media and scientific research. And while MS is indeed a game changer, it was my dear friend, comedian and fellow writer Tim Ferguson, who taught me that in devoting my (very precious) energy to something I love, I will always be able to push through the difficult days.

Just like one of my favourite quotes from John le Carre, "There's nothing so dangerous as a spy in a hurry"….. In writing the books as I do now, there is an urgency to tell stories and create content that might help people living with MS and their families make a paradigm shift from thinking that they're in a hopeless situation or that their life is over, to instead believing that the diagnosis of their condition could be something they can turn around into a positive. I hope that every reader will walk away with a couple more tricks to put in their toolbox so as they can live their life to the fullest; so that 'Taking Control' of a chronic illness is not only possible but empowering.

But my greatest wish in chronicling the lives of these nurses is that their selfless efforts and pursuits will be recognised and inspire action. Be that action for others to enter this tremendously vital – and by all accounts very satisfying – profession. Or that policy-makers and philanthropists globally will feel the impetus to support this profession because of the fundamentally positive effect a specialist nurse will have on nurturing their patient back into the fabric of society….. and often those people return to their lives more successfully, healthier or inherently as better human beings than before.

I'm a fervent advocate of storytelling to preserve our history, spark systemic change or ensure an enduring legacy. Storytelling has always been at the crux of my journalism career; it's what drives me and is my deep passion.

My journey throughout the creation of these books has been one of self-doubt to self-belief, anguish to elation, wonderment to outright indignation and all the time feeling a deep sense of commitment to get these stories right. To craft something that my subjects would be proud to hold up as a true representation of themselves for years to come. And whilst this is the last book in this particular series, I still feel the best is yet to some. I have never been happier and I can't wait for the next project to unfold.

Jillian Kingsford Smith

PS: Anyone who has ever been sick or is dealing with a chronic or life-threatening illness will know exactly the role nurses perform in their life. You can never repay them for the part they played in your recovery or in caring for your loved one.... Well, this is my way of saying thanks and acknowledging the difference they make in this world.

About the cover:

I ruminated and then agonised for some time in choosing the the cover image for this book. I wanted something immediately emblematic of nurses whilst also recognising that modern-day nursing doesn't necessitate a uniform. But then I was reminded of something Nicki Ward-Abel said in her interview:

"I have a theory that my uniform is representative of the line between nurse and patient. It allows me to listen and be empathetic and certainly feel everything I need to feel. But my uniform is also representative of the type of role I play in my patient's life and no matter how touched I am by my patients, I know the uniform gives me permission to go home at night and not carry their grief with me."

Upon further research, I came to understand that a fob watch or pendant watch is considered synonymous with nursing and that watches are sometimes given as a token rite-of-passage gift from parents to young nurses, who are making the transition into nurses' quarters and live away from home for the first time.

KAYE HOOPER
Queensland, Australia

*"You should go to university and study to be a doctor – we'll help
support you," my mum said to me.
"But mum I love being a nurse – I don't want to be a doctor."
And I knew it was as true then in 1980 as it is today in 2019.
But I am ahead of myself…*

I grew up in Sydney in the 1950s and 60s and I left school when I was fifteen years old after completing my School Certificate. I didn't really know what I wanted to do with my life, but when I started my nursing training a year later at Royal North Shore Hospital in Sydney, I knew I had found my life niche. After completing General Nursing, I started Midwifery Nurse training at King George V Hospital for Mothers and Babies in Sydney's Camperdown… and I loved it.

***

Learning about life and the world we live in.

Within six months of graduating from midwifery, I had become a Registered Midwife and Registered Nurse. Mum and dad were stoked as they really didn't know what I would do; let the adventures begin!

So, later that year, in 1974, I found myself sitting in a tiny, single prop plane which I'd boarded in Kano, Northern Nigeria in West Africa heading for a remote dirt airstrip next to a Mission Hospital in Sub Sahara Niger Republic. I was only just 21 and volunteering for a one-year stint alongside a small medical team; just one doctor and five nurses from UK, USA, Canada and Switzerland. I had no idea what I was in for!

It was hot all the time. This was a remote bush hospital in a barren landscape with no other medical facilities for hundreds of miles. The Hausas, Tuaregs and Bedouin peoples were our patients, brought to the hospital by camel, on foot, on a stretcher or oxen-drawn cart, covering their medical problem with a tattered cloth. It was sad, sad, sad.

That year was transformative for me in many ways; the ultimate juxtaposition to my life and work in Sydney. I delivered many babies in that west-African mission hospital and sadly most babies were not alive when the mother finally arrived at the hospital. This was because it was generally a two or three-day journey to get to us after many days of being in labour in small distant villages. The mothers were often young teenagers with their first pregnancy and had all the complications associated with that scenario. The year was full of massive stories and learning and I flew out of that village one year later, exhausted and wrung out, on my way to London before heading home to Australia.

I wasn't home in Australia for long before I was heading out to Africa again with the same mission, this time with another nurse who remains my close friend to this day. We were venturing across to re-start a small village clinic in South Sudan that had become deserted; a casualty of the long civil war. Finally, it was a time of peace and for two years we lived and worked in that small clinic and the village was our home. We were better prepared for life in

Africa this time. We delivered primary health care, vaccinations and basic emergency care to the Dinka and Nuer and Shilluk peoples of the Upper White Nile province. That was over forty years ago but amazingly – through social media – I have reconnected with many of my South Sudanese friends, who had become scattered around the world due to the more-recent African wars. Sadly, so many of our friends perished and the village was destroyed. Peace is still so fragile in 2019; restoration will take a long time.

Delivering health care in Africa was tricky. I learnt that when sick children weren't brought back to see us in the clinic, it was because the father had to plant next year's crops and it could take weeks to bring sick family members to us. Or is was because of other cultural morays that existed and restricted patient movements. And water to wash our hands before eating…really?? We insisted but we also saw the water that we washed our hands with over the dirt floor had been carried a kilometre on the head of a woman from the Nile swamp. Yes, it was complicated, and we learnt to appreciate the constraints and the culture that impacts health care provision.

I learnt a lot about life and the world we live in in my early twenties.

It was on my return from Africa back to Sydney that my mum suggested that I should "train to be a doctor" but I didn't want to; I just loved being a nurse: And still do today.

Back home again, I began my nursing career in research at the Royal Prince Alfred Hospital (RPAH). Clinical trials in perinatal research with hypertensive disease in pregnancy was my entrée. Then into Clinical Immunology and Allergy at RPWH and Sydney University. And it was then that I started studying for my Bachelor of Arts – my major in psychology – at Macquarie University in Sydney. I also did a grief counselling course, which upskilled me to better care for patients.

I worked in clinical immunology in Sydney for fourteen years and during this time I met my dear colleague Therese Burke who was doing similar work in clinical immunology at Westmead Hospital. What a joy it is to travel through my nursing career with treasured friends like Therese! There are great gifts in life and colleagues are one of them. I relocated to live and work in Brisbane in 1994 as part of Professor Pender's MS research team and then also became the MS Nurse Consultant at Royal Brisbane and Women's Hospital from 1996.

I had another overseas nursing stint in 2002, this time in Illinois in the United States for four years, and I was also able to slot into my nursing experiences the task of writing patient materials for the National MS Society in New York.

***

The Balancing Act

We take each of our roles in the MS process very seriously, and everyone in the process needs to understand they play a different role. As a nurse, I have a professional role, the patient is at the centre; and the role of the family or carer, which is different again... and in those early days after diagnosis, everyone is trying to work out their role. It's a bit like a jigsaw puzzle; we're all trying to work out where the gaps are, so we can insert our own particular expertise or areas of support.

Working as a MS nurse has changed my life in a lot of ways but one of the greatest things I've learned is to better balance life's uncertainties; I've learned to live the day at hand but still keep an eye on the future. And in many ways, that's exactly how I see my patients growing and changing their lives. Maybe it's because we actually live MS with them by proxy.

And in living with MS by proxy, sometimes if you're feeling vulnerable or tired or caught up in the middle of something terribly emotional and complex, it would be easy to feel a little non-committal to the patient in front of you. But first and foremost, it is our duty as MS nurses to approach each situation as if we are fresh. We may have just come out of a very difficult, confrontational or heart wrenching consultation; we may even feel worn down. But the minute I step out of my office door and greet the next person, you realise you've got to reset and give your next patient your 'bestest and freshest.' I can't say how we do it, I can't really provide any coping tactics; I just think as professionals we develop skills that allow us to compartmentalise and simply get on with things – even on those days when you've got a cracking headache or just had a lousy time even getting into the office. But the minute I start work I sequester that lousy thing that's bothering me and clear my head of my own story so as I can give the person sitting in front of me everything I have.

Is it a skill that's inherent in the type of people who become nurses? Probably. I personally draw a lot of energy from being with people and helping people, but conversely, I also like my alone time. As a whole though, being with people energises me and I learn and I love the conversations we have and luckily, only occasionally do you get fed up with the type of conversations being had!

When a patient asks me a question, the question itself will tell me where the person is at. For example, if a patient were to ask about alternative therapies, it might suggest to me that a family member or a friend is talking to them about steering clear of the disease modifying therapies (DMTs) and our traditional clinical options. Or perhaps there's something else in their head that is making them sceptical about the pharmaceutical treatments. If that is the first question that someone asks in their consultation, it is likely a priority for them at that time. And answering the question is key at that point, so as the patient can concentrate on everything else.

And no matter whether you agree with the area of concern being put forward, if you don't address those issues then you really aren't meeting their needs. There really is nothing more you need to do than work your way through the topic and as you do, I often find you'll take detours based on the patient's further probing or when it becomes obvious that the patient is unaware or unclear of the explanation you're providing.

And really, the more we can explain about the disease itself, how the symptoms may manifest, and all the facets of treatment and symptom management, then we're helping demystify the condition and it hopefully becomes a little less scary. And particularly when we can make MS become more personal and individual – that's when I start to see a better level of comprehension as the information sinks in.

Consultations and interactions with my patients are definitely a balancing act. It's imperative to listen and understand where people are at, but I also need to be able to read between the lines whilst trying to contain the tangents of conversation that get thrown up... those out of the blue queries or remarks that will want to explore the minutia of the disease or the irrationalities of it all. Sometimes it's just not helpful to over-examine everything all at once.

And sometimes I think patients just don't know exactly what to ask, so instead they'll ask something a little esoteric or obtuse. And in those times where we'll end up a bit off-topic or in a confused and convoluted conversation, I'll reset the consultation by simply asking "is there a question I'm not asking that you think I should?"

During my consultations – and in fact throughout most people's disease course – I generally know what questions I'm likely to be asked, but also what I'll need to ask of my patient. Although if it's ME who's confused about the topic of conversation (and it's easy to understand how confusion arises when we're talking about the many and varied aspects of MS) I'll need to try and work out what it really is that we're talking about so as I can provide better information and support. If the patient is still a bit confused or wafty, a good strategy I'll use is to say "well, some people at this point might ask me this…." And because I've heard at least a million questions over the course of my twenty five years of being a MS nurse I'll be able to get to the bottom of what my patient really wants to explore.

It takes time and experience but as a MS nurse, you do learn that skill of interpreting what is really bothering people at any given point.

Another common challenge during a consultation might be when the person living with MS has brought a family member along. And it's something we generally encourage, but you can easily multiply the number of questions by three! In these situations, I prefer to face and talk directly to the patient, whilst knowing that their relatives are listening to the conversation. And I also find with several people in the room, you just have to take one thing at a time. Some of the questions may end up being rehashed consultation-after-consultation, especially while the patient or their family make the various adjustments to living with MS; and sometimes it's a case of having to answer the same question in a variety of ways to compensate for different communication or comprehension levels.

And the questions are pretty consistent across a multitude of conditions. They're the immediate, big, scary, rest-of-life questions such as:

- Can I give this to my kids?
- Will I die from this?
- Will I end up in a wheelchair?
- Can I continue with my work or career?

And then you start transitioning into the logistical or applied questions like:
- Who do I need to tell at work?
- Do I need to tell anyone at all?
- What happens to my insurance?
- Should I do this or should I do that?

But really and truly it's all too much to take in right after you've been told you have multiple sclerosis. I prefer to explain that I'm going to take the person on a trip a bit like a 'highlights of Europe' trip that takes 21 days. We're going to see a little bit of everything, but you have to know that you'll want to come back and visit the stuff that really interests you later on. And not to be worried, because you WILL be able to revisit... multiple times if necessary.

A broad sweep of information is about the only thing you can offer in those early sessions and being able to judge the pace that people can handle is a really essential skill to cultivate. And how people absorb information and learn is the other side of this process: How do people twig to the material you're providing? Some people may be nodding in acceptance, but I can generally tell if it's not the case at all. It's then I might go into explaining the same thing in two different ways – ensuring one way is visual and the other way is descriptive, or perhaps one explanation is laden with details and references and another way might be a bit more global and generic. It's a case of working out where people are at emotionally and psychologically, and this can take time in simply getting to know patients; knowing how to connect with them and what resonates. And also working out if there's other things they're dealing with apart from the MS, such as financial burden or spousal problems or challenges with their children. Sometimes the MS is so secondary to everything else.

***

Thoroughbreds and brumbies

Clinical trials are nearly always conducted with what I call 'pristine people.' People who are the 'thoroughbreds' of the research world because they don't have many other (or excluded) anomalies. Their age fits within a certain range, their health is largely good in specific areas and they have the time for a clinical trial, so they likely have less constraints at home.

But in our regular outpatient clinics, we're dealing with 'brumbies' every day. In fact, most people in life are brumbies – let's face it! And patients participating in clinical trials and research are just so important to what we do, but when it comes to interpreting information and facts and variables whilst sitting face-to-face with our patients, you need time, knowledge and understanding and compassion and experience. I am grateful for the statistics and epidemiology I learnt in my Master of Public Health course – to decipher and help explain treatment outcomes to my patients.

You can't just give medicine or advice in a vacuum. It's my role to figure out what else is going on in my patient's life so I can best support them. Take for instance if they're homeless or financially burdened. They're unlikely to take medicine or adhere to treatment. And this is why you also need a team approach to MS. Some people don't need a lot of help to navigate MS but there are others who need every bit of help you can give. In our clinic environment, we need to be aware of the general things that go on in life and have a team who can each do their part to support the person with MS.

I imagine it could be quite frustrating for people with MS in those early days, when they're trying to come to terms with their many and varying symptoms. The literature on the web will explain the most common of symptoms and give a bit of an idea on how someone might feel. But something I find myself explaining to my patients is that this information is based off studies that by necessity need to generalise the findings. So, for someone experiencing sensation issues in their arm, it could range from a mild tingling sensation right though to an extreme numbness. And it could be fleeting or permanent. Apply that across some twenty symptoms that are deemed 'common' in MS and it is overwhelming.

Now let's layer a treatment over the top of that mixed bag; a treatment that provides hope to dampening some of the disease activity of MS, but again, it's been trialled on a many and varied cohort of people and at this time we can't distinguish who will get the most benefit and who won't. As we discover more about MS, we will be able to tailor treatments to individual needs. It's no wonder people with MS get frustrated when they can't pinpoint what's going on and for how long. I want to guide my patients through this time to give them clarity on what we do know and ask them to be positive and hopeful for the future.

Sometimes I wake up in the middle of the night wondering if I've ordered a particular test or sent out some material or what have you. I learned a little trick years ago called the 'peg system.' It helps me remember tasks for easy recall and by doing this, I find I can quickly get the tasks off my mind and chase a bit of rest. And that's not to say that other things – particularly medical things – don't also worry me but I'd like to think that I do enough cross-checking and talking with colleagues to make sure I've covered off everything medically.

It is important that my patients and their families don't blame everything on MS. It's very easy to think that MS is causing every little ache, anomaly or mishap in your body, but to do that could detract from other health concerns that may be occurring. As nurses, we want to make sure the entire medical team – from the neurologist to the GP to the physiotherapists and allied health professionals – are coaching our patients to live as healthily as possible. And it's worth mentioning here that the general practitioner has a crucial role in the care of people with MS.

One of the things I like to differentiate MS from is something like a stroke. I think when someone is newly diagnosed with MS, they believe they're going to experience – or keep experiencing – these big moments where they're struck down with a MS attack. I like to explain that MS is not usually an emergency disease. Mostly with MS, people will deal with MS relapses that come on slowly, cause a problem for a length of time, then it may improve, or it may just wobble along for a bit. But rarely anymore do we see MS striking people down and causing immediate locked-in effects the way a stroke might.

***

As MS nurses, one of our primary roles within the clinical team dynamic is to endeavour to spend the time with our patients; as much time as possible. It's our job to understand what the patient is asking and it's our job to help the patient learn about the condition they're living with. It's our job to be there for our patients and advocate for them with others whenever needed.

And in that way, the role the MS nurse plays is integral. There's been so many studies that show when a person is first diagnosed with just about any type of chronic condition and meets with a specialist and a nurse, so little of the initial information actually sinks in. And understandably so. These generally unsuspecting people find themselves in a new world with new medical language that they have to understand and it's hard going. It's our job to help pick up the pieces later and make sure the information registers.

And in those early appointments post-diagnosis, you can absolutely be given too much information that may never be relevant to you – ever! While we know there's some commonalities in MS, most people just have to live life for a while – and see what is going to be relevant to them – as time goes on. And it's the feeling of uncertainty that is very scary to people. They may constantly wonder what's going to happen next? Will anything at all happen next? Should they ring a doctor or a nurse because of something odd that they're feeling? How should they feel at any given point in time? How will they feel when or if something does happen? That constant fear and feedback loop becomes a real problem.

For a lot of patients, the biggest support we can provide is to simply reassure that help is at hand; that I am on the end of a phone line; that they are not alone. And sometimes I can't solve any definitive problems, but I can at least listen to them or let them know if something sounds 'normal' and isn't worth worrying about. I have a lot of conversations that start off with people saying "Kaye, this might sound a bit strange but…" But nothing sounds strange any longer; I have heard it all!

***

My career has encompassed two quite long-term positions that simultaneously involved research duties and clinical care. It's actually quite uncommon to experience this and I'm tremendously grateful as I've loved the wonderful combination.

If you forge a career in research – and you're lucky enough to be involved in world-class research – then it means you're with a group of people who are serious about good medicine and serious about solving a problem intellectually. The sharp minds that I've had the privilege to work with are truly inspiring. And the research I've worked in was not pharmaceutical-driven research but instead sought the cause of MS. It was very exciting but also very, very practical.

And the other thing that is a bit different about my career trajectory is that I've never worked in the wards, because I spent all that time in Africa and then went down the path of clinical and research roles. I've had as much patient-facing experience as anyone, but within different environments.

When I think about my collective career experiences, I never went into anything feeling overconfident, but I knew I wanted to at least give things a go. I didn't want the opportunity to pass me by.... embracing the unknown and following the adventure were definitely the driving forces behind anything I chose to do.

The director of the Neuro-immunology Research Centre at the University of Queensland, Professor Michael Pender, asked me to take up the role of MS Nurse Consultant and Manager when he established the MS Clinic at RBWH in 1996 to coincide with the first MS treatment becoming available in Australia. It was at this time that I felt I needed to establish some connections with other experienced MS nurses who could support and guide me in what I was about to embark on.

Specialist nursing can be a bit isolating at times because it's not as if there's a lot of you running around in the one place! So, in my holiday time I decided to meet some of the MS Nurses I had contacted in

USA and was encouraged to attend a Consortium of MS Centres (CMSC) meeting in 1997 in Calgary, Canada. It was there I met June Halper – and a number of other colleagues who remain dear friends today – and together we became the founding members of the International Organization of MS Nurses (IOMSN).

The mission of the IOMSN was to establish and perpetuate a specialised branch of nursing in multiple sclerosis; to establish standards of nursing care in multiple sclerosis; to support multiple sclerosis nursing research; and to educate the health care community about multiple sclerosis and to disseminate this knowledge throughout the world.

But the ultimate goal of the IOMSN was to improve the lives of all those persons affected by multiple sclerosis through the provision of appropriate healthcare services and to make hope happen!

June had brought a lawyer along to formalise the organisation and from this we formed a management board, on which I sat for a number of years.

So I returned to Australia enthusiastic and focussed on starting an Australian group. In 1998, with the help of MS nurse researcher Judy Wollin, we set up the MS Nurses Australia (MSNA). Soon after we included our New Zealand colleagues as well, becoming MS Nurses Australasia. MSNA became an official affiliate with IOMSN.

We realised that our organisation needed to be formally incorporated, which required some guidance from a lawyer. As it happened, I was walking along a city street in Brisbane soon after my return from Calgary, talking to a colleague and saw a sign for a lawyer's office and thought 'why not?' So up I walked into this lawyer's office and explained the situation of needing to form an incorporated association for MS nurses. He informed us his best friend was living with MS and he offered to help us pro bono. How wonderful his help was.

Both organisations have gone from strength to strength for our nursing community, and worldwide there have been many MS Nurse organisations established. Such a great resource for us all, as we share information and experiences and as patients move around the world and resettle, it is a delight to let them know the name of their 'new MS Nurse' in their new country.

We now have an international certification process and exam, which was borne from the desire to set an international standard on the basic principles of MS and its management, treatment and research.

The Multiple Sclerosis Nurses International Certification Board (MSNICB) was established by the IOMSN to develop criteria for certification and re-certification and administer the Certification Examination for Multiple Sclerosis Nurses. The IOMSN endorses the concept of voluntary certification by examination for nursing professionals providing care in multiple sclerosis. Those who work or have worked in this specialty and meet eligibility requirements may be candidates to take this examination.

Certification focuses specifically on the individual and is an indication of knowledge and skills in MS practice. MS nursing certification provides normal recognition of a level of knowledge in the field and promotes delivery of safe and effective practice in the domains of Clinical Practice (disease course and epidemiology of MS, pathology, diagnosis, pharmacologic therapies, non-pharmacologic therapies, psychosocial assessment and interventions),

Advocacy (ethical practice, negotiating the healthcare system, empowerment, knowledge of the community resources, patient rights, consultation expertise); Education (principles of teaching/learning, health promotion and change theory, special populations professional development); and Research (evidence based practice, protection of human subjects, research terminology and process).

The exam is offered to potential candidates in IOMSN member countries at least once a year, and whilst not mandatory for employment in the world, the credential has now become highly regarded as a best-practice indicator.

***

Sometimes it is what it is...

I have learnt from so many people and so many different places over my lifetime. I've been a specialist MS nurse for more than twenty-five years, and nursing for nearly 50 years. So in that time I've talked to a lot of neurologists, specialists, researchers, other MS nurses and of course, patients.

But it is my patients I've known over the years that have filled my life, pulled my heart, broadened my parameters and inspired me. I've met people from all walks of life in different places and times and circumstances. My landscape in the field of MS is forever filling out.

MS nursing is an adventure, unpredictable – a bit 'messy' – because every day and every task, every interaction is different. Just as every person we meet is different and every person living with MS has a unique MS experience. For those diagnosed with MS it is a lifelong experience. As nurses we get to know our patients sometimes when they are students at university, studying; applying for jobs, getting married, having children, travelling, getting older, dealing with other medical issues…and MS tags along in all these stages. I love it that we get to see the baby photos and the wedding photos and the awards achieved. The nurse/patient relationships can last a long time and are precious!

And for me, the simple act of listening has been one of the most valuable ways I learn. From listening to people and hearing their experiences and being part of the problem-solving process. I've learned that listening is a massively vital part of our role as a MS nurse.

A lot of people want to tell you stuff, but they don't want to listen.

Say you go out to dinner and a friend will tell you a story about how they had a disastrous holiday, they missed their plane and then suffered delays. And immediately you're thinking about the time you missed a plane and you want to tell your story and then you're no longer listening to your friend's story.

So I think – as nurses – we learn to sit and listen so we know best how to help. And then you realise a lot more about yourself. Things like how your own stories can get in the way and how you can't listen properly. I'm not saying it isn't hard; we are human after all – but we all do it.

Back in 1990 when I was working in Sydney, I worked with people who had pregnancy loss. Many patients talked to me about sadness and difficult life experiences and I knew I needed to do some grief counselling education. At the course, one of the key things I learned was to not let your own story get in the way and instead simply listen and hear what people are saying.

One memorable lesson from 1990s was from the husband of a

patient. He was standing in the rain outside his house, speaking to me on the phone about another miscarriage his wife had endured. It was heartbreaking, and after he finished his story I remember being full of so many emotions and I simply said "I don't know what to say…"

His reply is still clear to me decades later. He replied "Thank you for listening. There really is nothing to say."

The lesson I took from that exchange is that listening is powerful and comforting; it's a gesture to the patient that signifies they are not alone. Not everything we hear as nurses is something that needs to be fixed. Sometimes it is what it is. A person telling you a simple fact. A fact that doesn't need solving or alleviating. It merely needs acknowledgement.

And that can be a hard one for nurses, because there's an inherent sense that we need to fix things and sometimes you just can't. But I know we'll still be wanting to fix things and questioning ourselves as to whether we did enough!

Over the course of my career I've certainly sat in a consulting room or talking on the phone with some very unhappy people – sometimes because of poorly chosen words or misunderstandings. These are difficult situations. It may have started out after a previous conversation with another member of the team that went poorly or another interaction with other staff in the hospital. Repairing these interpersonal relationships is complicated. There's a lot of reflection after these situations where we need to examine what we could have done better, and a great deal of the time there's other factors at play. It's not simply that wrong words were said. It may be something completely separate that the patient is experiencing at home and they've brought that problem into the clinic. Or it could be a specialist who hasn't been given the entire story from the patient… either way, they can be very hard situations to remedy.

And sometimes a particular nurse/patient relationship is just not a good fit. It might never be a good fit, or it might not be a good fit at that moment in time. With the passage of time, a person living with MS will experience changes. Their view on life or the disease or how they interact with those around them – all this will change.

And that change a person experiences over time when living with MS is really crucial for both the nurse and the patient to note. But particularly for the patient…. I'll often hear from a newly diagnosed person that in those first few years they'll wake up and tentatively do a body scan, trying to assess what works and what doesn't that day. And that can be a very nervous way to wake up every day.

But over time, people build a confidence that they will be able to manage with most things that the day brings. Or they become attuned at living with the uncertainty because they know how to set limits on their energy or body or the conditions they put themselves under each day. And then everyone is different and then you can also go through good phases and bad phases and ups and downs. And it comes back to my other point about teasing out the issues or even just letting something 'be' for a bit. These are all strategies we need in our nurse's tool kit to help a patient and also minimise those moments where we wonder 'what more could I have done?'

***

Building your 'nurse muscles.'

We live with the knowledge that we can't fix everything. We need a cure; we need to be able to repair the damage and we need to find a way to stop MS from occurring. Until that time, we live with things that are not fixable. Yes there are treatments and management strategies to alleviate some of the symptoms but I know that there's an enormous number of people living with MS who are living life well. I hear from many of my patients that they have seen life in new ways and no longer sweat the small things and the joys of life are richer. They absolutely have good days and bad days, but by their own admission, many are living far better lives than at pre-diagnosis and they're doing so with a disease we can't yet cure. So there can be a middle ground for both nurses and patients to appreciate in finding joy in the yet unfixable life of MS.

The things that stick in my mind are the conversations with patients where they just demonstrate how well they're coping or how they choose to look at things in a positive light. The patients who tell you that being in a wheelchair means they get the best seats at a concert or that being diagnosed has allowed them to redesign their life to be far better. I have written letters to employers of my patients with medical requests for a change of hours or a tweak in the working environment. This is so positive because most of my patients want to remain working and feeling fulfilled and they just need to make some small modifications to do so. These are the people who just want to get on with living. It's really cool and their stories give me a lot of joy.

I often reflect how becoming a MS nurse has provided me the opportunities to increase my professional skills and certainly my personal skills in ways I didn't know possible. As nurses, we're put in such a wide variety of situations with a multitude of different people with different characteristics and different demeanours. And learning how to read and cope with each of those variances allows you to build what I call 'nurse muscles.' And those muscles are the ones you develop because you have to do a lot of things you've never ever had to do before. You basically live MS with the person you're helping and people with MS are really not experiencing anything much different to what we go through as nurses. Most of them can relate to our journey in life because they're obviously living it too. Just as we've built 'nurse muscles' they've built 'MS muscles.'

And in that way, I think many people living with MS show wisdom and strength because they've learned that life has thrown up challenges and difficulties. They've had to speed up learning a lot of life skills and adjust to challenges as they face the ups and downs of the bumpy road of MS.

For me, being a MS Nurse has been a rich and rewarding vocation, learning and participating in research and delivering health care to many. I am grateful for my colleagues who have propped me up when I felt down and laughed and cheered me on in celebrating the good times. Most of all it is a privilege to share in a patient's life journey. And patients have also inspired me with their strength and courage to face the day, to get on with life – even if a physical strength is lacking.

So is there one word to describe how I feel about what I do? I would have the say the word 'delighted' is the first word that pops into my head. Followed very closely by the word 'privileged.'

But I just love being a nurse!

My hopes for the future treatment and management of MS:

•   Finding a cure. I hope there will be some way to stop the disease from starting in the first place. But that means we need to know the mechanism for how it starts. And I guess that's the precise reason for the work we're doing with Professor Pender.

•   Treatment to repair the damage already done to regain and recover function.

•   Identification of the people who are at risk genetically for developing MS. Then having a vaccination to stop them getting MS.

•   Discovering and refining the management of MS symptoms. Maybe it's because we better understand the symptoms and complexity of MS and how it affects so much of a person. But to me, it's very encouraging that we can help people live a better life because we clinically understand far more about those symptoms now.

•   There should be more MS Nurses available for patients in the health care system – to help and support patients as needed.

My advice for nurses beginning their career:

•   The world of MS holds many challenging and interesting opportunities for MS Nurses.

•   Listen more and talk less when you are with patients.

•   Make sure the patient knows how to navigate their health care system and who to contact.

- Reassure the patient that they are not alone and help is near.

- Learn the basics of MS – build up your medical and scientific knowledge and keep up to date.

- Try to get involved in research – it's fascinating and exciting work.

- Learn from other MS nurses and set up your own network of peer support.

- Look after yourself. When you need a break, take time out and learn to debrief with a colleague or counsellor.

- Caring for a patient with MS is a team effort and the MS Nurse is an important member of the team.

- Enjoy it and embrace every opportunity to learn and grow in the role.

- Respect a patient's decision. Discuss decisions openly and review management plans regularly. Every decision we make does not have to be forever.

- Reassure the patient that when you make a decision, just know why you made the decision. Because when you look back, you will be clear as to the various factors that influenced your decision-making. And that's not to say that a decision can't be reviewed or changed later as the circumstances change.

JUNE HALPER

New Jersey, Unites States of America

*"We have to keep reminding ourselves why we're in the business.
We're in this to take care of people with MS. And what matters most
to them should matter most to us."*

The greatest advance in the treatment of MS I've seen over the course of my career has been the emergence of the MS nurse. Nearly four decades ago when I started, there was maybe four of us around, and now we have hundreds of MS nurses all over the world. To me, that's the most significant advancement.

Having said that, becoming a MS nurse was strictly an accident for me! At the time, there was no intention of consciously pursuing a career in MS. I go back to 1978 when, as a young nurse, I was undertaking further studies in public health and had returned to college.

During this, I had to find an agency or a position for three months that met the needs of the curriculum for the advanced degree in public health and somewhere I could also develop health programmes and resources. I was fully intending to do the residency and move on with my studies, but some 39 years later I'm still here working in MS! I fell in love with my patients and the daily challenges I was presented, so there was really never any question that I would leave.

Back in those earlier days of working in public health and before I began my residency, many of the people I had seen who were living with MS were patients who were quite progressed and often confined to their homes. At the time I thought everyone diagnosed with multiple sclerosis was bed-bound and weathering bed sores. It probably didn't help that the catchcry of the MS Society was "MS: The crippling disease of young adults."

But only a few years later when I went into that residency with MS patients, I got to meet people who would walk into our centre, and many of them didn't need wheelchairs and were still working and clearly not disabled, as I'd previously perceived the entire cohort of people living with MS to be. I realised that the spectrum of MS was much different to what was being publicised by the MS Society at the time. I quickly came to understand that it was beneficial for fundraising activities to call MS a 'crippling' disease and to show people in wheelchairs. But also, this was back in the early '80s when there certainly wasn't as much to offer people with MS either, so the outlook was a little more challenging than what we know today.

I've always steadfastly leaned towards the philosophy of wellness and empowerment. But let's face it, back when I started in MS over forty years ago, the best we could offer our patients by way of support was simply ourselves. There wasn't a lot of specific information or resources about MS we could equip ourselves with. The variety of treatments and level of research and knowledge of how to manage the disease just wasn't there like it is now.

So by the time I was fully immersed in MS nursing in the '80s, I realised how much there was to be done. It was clear that a much higher level of education and awareness was needed to change that dire perception of people living with MS as being crippled and disabled. It was also obvious to me that the comprehensive care model was the right way to go and adopting this philosophy would provide a far greater outcome for those people and their families affected by MS. I could see that it was very difficult for a neurologist to manage holistic MS patient care all by themselves. The role of the nurse or the rehabilitation specialist was also a vital piece of the puzzle.

And that was when I started to work with a team to develop a heads of care centre in New Jersey.

In 1985 we finally opened the MS Center at the Holy Name Medical Center in Teaneck New Jersey. The MS clinic later became the Alfiero and Lucia Pelestroni Foundation Multiple Sclerosis Center in 2018 to honour a generous donation from the Palestroni Foundation.

Within twelve months of opening the MS clinic in New Jersey, a number of neurologists – led by Dr. Donald Taty in Canada – got together with the view to forming a consortium of MS specialists; I was invited to join that founding group.

Organised in 1986 under the direction of neurologists and specialists dedicated to the clinical care of MS, the Consortium of Multiple Sclerosis Centers (CMSC) has evolved into a multi -disciplinary organisation providing a team approach to MS care and a network for all health care professionals and related specialists in the care of persons with MS.

The CMSC is now the largest organisation of multiple sclerosis health professionals in North America and certainly one of the most distinguished centres for MS care globally. Since its inception, the

CMSC has grown to over 250-member centres in the United States, Canada, South America, and Europe, and represents over 12,000 health care professionals worldwide who provide care for more than 250,000 individuals with MS and their families.

The CMSC includes numerous individual members who are neurologists, nurses, psychologists, and rehabilitation professionals. It has members who are academic centers, community programs, veterans affairs medical centers, individual healthcare providers, students, corporate sponsors, and non-profit partners such as LACTRIMS (the Latin American counterpart of the CMSC) and RIMS (the European counterpart) providing comprehensive care in multiple sclerosis.

From the outset, the vision of the CMSC was to become the pre-eminent organisation of MS professionals. The team sought to achieve this through collaborative and interdisciplinary approaches, and by leading the development and dissemination of scientifically based knowledge regarding MS clinical care. The ultimate goal was – and remains – to improve the lives of those affected by multiple sclerosis.

To that end, the CMSC engages in activities that consist of professional education, clinical research, advocacy, and communication of activities to the healthcare community. CMSC is particularly interested in the future of chronic care and the role of alternative care in the 21st century.

I was a member of the consortium representing the MS clinic at the Holy Name Center for a number of years. Then around 1990 the consortium decided to form a board, of which I took on the treasurer's role. And I knew how to undertake that role like I knew how to perform brain surgery, but I happily took on the role regardless! Then in 1992 there was a reorganisation of the Consortium and I was delegated to the secretariat's role for a couple of months. Well those few months turned into quite a long time and some thirty years later I'm still here! I eventually served as the consortium's president from 1995 to 1997 and have also been its CEO since 1992.

Who knew that a seemingly inconsequential residency back in 1978 would lead into such immersive experiences as developing the MS Center in New Jersey and then being at the coalface of the enormous impact of the CMSC? And I was about to add another dimension to my collective experiences with the formation of the first and only international organisation focusing solely on the needs and goals of professional multiple sclerosis nurses.

It was 1997 and I'd been invited to attend a pharmaceutical conference about emerging disease modifying therapies (DMTs) in Calgary, Canada. I met an Australian nurse named Kaye Hooper. She'd paid for herself to come all the way over as she was desperate to meet other nurses in the field of MS and learn from them and share experiences. Both Kaye and I got to talking and realised that there was an inherent need for nurses all over the world to have a 'home;' a place where they could meet and talk and network, become mentored and fine-tune their education. That very night we mapped out the formation of the International Organisation of Multiple Sclerosis Nurses (IOMSN).

The mission of the IOMSN was to the establish and perpetuate a specialised branch of nursing in multiple sclerosis; to establish standards of nursing care in multiple sclerosis; to support multiple sclerosis nursing research; and to educate the health care community about multiple sclerosis and to disseminate this knowledge through-out the world.

But the ultimate goal of the IOMSN is to improve the lives of all those persons affected by multiple sclerosis through the provision of appropriate healthcare services and to make hope happen!

***

"All of a sudden, MS became a very treatable disease."

I know many, many people criticise the pharmaceutical companies and scepticism of their social conscience runs deep, but a great deal of our progress with this disease over the years has to do with the development and introduction of the DMTs. As nurses and rehabilitation specialists and physical therapists, we could very ably assist in managing MS symptoms and monitoring the mental health of our patients, but that real turning point was when we started seeing patients on DMTs such as Betaferon, Copaxone and Rebif, and later on with Tysabri. All those early treatments coming onto market made a huge difference in the lives of people living with MS but also the work we did as nurses.

All of a sudden MS became a very treatable disease. And once we started seeing MS as a treatable disease, we started educating our patients on the benefits of exercise and healthy lifestyles. And once people started recognising their disease's treatability, they also recognised the value in forming a comprehensive care team that incorporated modalities such as physical and rehabilitation therapy, mental health specialists, clinical specialists, complementary medicine and of course, MS nursing.

And basically at the CMSC, we work with our patients to form their 'A team,' and I couldn't be more excited that this comprehensive care approach is being recognised worldwide as a best-practice in treating MS. Importantly, I see our role as MS nurses as coordinating this A-team under the leadership of the patient. We help the patient assemble their own team, which might include a neurologist, physiotherapist, general practitioner, psychologist and even right down to finding the appropriate people in the community who can help them with group exercise programmes, support groups or social activities. We like to think of it as creating a holistic package of wellness.

Years ago, the biggest challenge for people with MS was that they were being told 'don't have kids, quit your job, in fact, just don't do too much at all.' Now we know all of that is bad advice. Decades ago when you were diagnosed you were basically told to go home and live with MS and just call in if you had a problem. I know anecdotally there were people with MS contemplating suicide because they didn't know what else to do.

Today, the message is, and needs to be continually reinforced, as being the polar opposite. Our message as MS nurses is to implore our patients not to give up; as specialist nurses we need to do everything we can to help our patients live and stay well and do things that normalise their life. We know now that exercise helps sustain brain plasticity and these are far better images and messages to get across to people living with MS. No longer should the disease be seen as one where people are wheelchair bound.

And the other thing I advocate very loudly for in people diagnosed with MS is that MS shouldn't become their career. There is nothing more boring than being so consumed by a chronic condition that it defines you. You don't want to make MS who you are. It's certainly part of who you are – like it or not – but it should only be a small facet of what you are.

I only stopped practicing as a 'hands on' MS nurse quite recently: But I don't think we ever stop 'being' a MS nurse! I still keep in touch with many of my patients and they still reach out with various questions and call me for advice, but I don't treat them any longer. Mostly they want to know what's new in the world of MS research. And there's so many wonderful things we can now talk about.

When I first started as a MS nurse, one of the biggest challenges for me was the sadness I'd experience when patients passed away. Again, this was before the introduction of the effective treatments that are now available. Simply put, people without treatment didn't do well. But these days, we know that people passing away from MS was a phenomenon and we have many great DMTs available and people can live long and full lives with MS. However, thirty and forty years ago, they were dying of complications of being unhealthy whilst living with MS, obviously not from the MS itself. The message of being able to live a healthy life whilst managing MS wasn't even really a thing.

If I had a patient who passed away from complications I'd almost feel like a failure. But these were patients who were in full-time nursing care, dealing with respiratory complications and the like, and their own families could no longer give them the support they needed. Thankfully, these days we just don't see that happen very often at all. We see fewer wheelchairs, we see much fewer cases of extreme disability. The outlook is much better for someone diagnosed now.

But one thing the development of the new DMTs has taken away from us is the concept of time. By that, I mean with the earlier pharmaceutical treatments, we might spend five years and more trialling the drugs. These earlier treatments may or may not have lacked the sophistication of some of the DMTs we have available now, but we certainly knew how people were doing five and ten years plus after being on these treatments. There's no denying that with something like Tysabri and Copaxone, we have collected mountains of information and have a great deal of clarity around their side effects and efficacy. But the newer DMTs, for as wonderful as they are, we lack that longer-term knowledge of how people are faring decades down the track.

I'm hoping that due to the seriousness of these newer treatments, the trials will start to extend out again. And I say that knowing that people living with MS want – and deserve – to have highly effective treatments as soon as possible. But I'd just like to see a bit more research… We really need longer ranging data on these newer DMTs to fully understand if their benefits hold. To put it simply, if the risk is worth the reward.

Regardless, it's still an extremely exciting time to be a MS nurse. And even for someone diagnosed with MS today you could say that it's a good time to be living with MS.

***

"I think the cure – or at least an ideology of a cure – is certainly coming."

Despite my pontification about the trialling of treatments and better determining the long- term benefits, getting patients diagnosed faster and onto the most beneficial treatment for them is one of the most exciting things I'm seeing in MS.

Even with the development and formal acknowledgement of RIS – radiologically isolated syndrome – we're seeing patients who have gone in for an MRI to have headaches examined and the MRI is picking up MS disease activity. Neurologists may now choose to start patients on MS treatments based on those types of MRI findings. The new McDonald criteria of 2017 has been amended to include the findings of the initial MRI as an acceptable diagnosis of MS. Prior to this, if a person had numbness and tingling down their legs combined with activity on the MRI they couldn't count that MRI sign as a diagnosis but would instead have to wait for the lesion to become further symptomatic and several attacks or flares to occur.

The latest revisions to the McDonald criteria enable neurologists to determine a diagnosis after a single MS event. And still do so comprehensively. With this, a patient can now be diagnosed earlier and started on a therapy if they choose, which would generally benefit the entire disease course of a patient greatly. I live in immense hope that people won't have to wait months or even years to be certain about their diagnosis but instead able to start the process of finding the most appropriate treatment.

The second thing I hope for is that someone, someday, will figure out what causes or triggers MS. Just think then about how we might be able to create targeted treatments if we knew more about the cause... Diagnosis would very likely be a faster process and even disease prevention might be possible.

And whilst talking about causes, I think there's a lot of optimism around studying the genetics of MS so that we can personalise the treatments to the symptoms. I look at the great things that scientists are doing within the field of cancer research and genetics and the possibility of targeting gene therapies for the treatment of MS is exciting to me.

I started my story by stating that the greatest advance in the treatment of MS I've seen over the course of my career has been the emergence of the MS nurse. This definite shift to having the advanced practice nurse so intrinsically involved in the patient's treatment protocol is incredibly significant. It's a positive allocation of resources, alleviating the pressure from the neurologist yet still providing the person living with MS much readier access to an integral specialist.

And now that we have a growing collegiate of MS nurses, it means we all have greater resources in each other to lean on and support one another, both personally and professionally. This again benefits the MS community.

I've noticed there's a serious sense of awe that a patient experiences when talking to their neurologist. In fact, I'm sure there's been a tonne of studies done on this very phenomenon! But there's also a serious dichotomy in how this 'awe' confounds the MS patient and they either don't hear what the neurologist is saying, or they may be too embarrassed to ask questions or confide the level of personal information they should.

So I find it really useful to speak with patients after a neuro consult. I begin by asking them how the appointment was and what they understood the neuro to have recommended? The comfort level with a neurologist or specialist physician is often not the same as what you would have with a nurse. Generally my patients will confide they were too embarrassed to ask the neuro to clarify various points of the suggested treatments or explain what a clinical finding meant. However, they have a different bond – a different relationship – with the nurse and feel like they can speak in plain language and ask for an explanation in plain language.

You can easily gauge the value that is placed on the role of the MS nurse when you take a look at how many nurses are being swayed to work for pharmaceutical companies. Big pharma knows how important that nurse/patient relationship is. And having those nurses and health care professionals work between the neurologists and MS nurses in our clinic and the scientists at the pharmaceutical companies is fairly beneficial too. It's great for keeping the channels of communication open amongst all the stakeholders. Free-flowing dialogue again, can only benefit the patient.

***

"Grant me the serenity to accept the things I cannot change."

It's very hard – particularly for someone in their twenties – to be confronted with a chronic illness. As a person grows older (like it or hate it) it's more usual to find something wrong or just be more reconciled with the aging process. And I guess that's the first challenge to accept; that you may have a chronic illness for the rest of your life but it needs to integrate into everything else you have going on, all without becoming so consumed by it that it becomes your career.

Then you have to develop something that we don't normally have to develop until we get a bit older, which is a wellness lifestyle. In our teens and twenties, we tend to take our health for granted; we consider ourselves invulnerable and bullet proof. But then suddenly you find yourself with a disease that can potentially affect you in just about every single part of your body. And to be able to learn how to stay well with all that going on takes some skill. As strange as it is to point out, I believe that being diagnosed with MS can be a blessing for some people. Because by the time we think about adopting a wellness lifestyle normally, you may have already developed obesity or habits with food and alcohol or poor mental health. Taking a good hard look at how you'll healthily and sustainably live your life can only be a good thing and the earlier that is done, the better.

Ultimately accepting the uncertainty of living with a chronic disease is also something that benefits people with MS. It would scare the pants off me, but if you can, get your mind around the uncertain nature of MS sooner rather than later.

And there are things in MS you can control – like minimising stress, getting the right kind of exercise, eating well and getting enough rest – but having a relapse is not necessarily something that you can control. But you simply can not live in fear every day that you'll relapse. It's almost like the line from AA's 12 Steps programme.

*"Grant me the serenity to accept the things I cannot change.
Courage to change the things I can.
And the Wisdom to know the difference."*

I think the worst part of living with uncertainty is not knowing if or when another relapse will come, how severe it might be or what damage it may do. I'm reminded of a study I read recently that found with today's DMTs we're still not teaching patients what a relapse actually is. In some cases, patients will be under the impression that because they're taking one of these wonderful treatments, that they'll never experience a relapse. The study shows that many relapses experienced by MS patients go unreported.

Despite the desire to have my patients embrace the notion of accepting the things they can't change, I still personally find it difficult to accept there are some things I can't help with either. Unfortunately, I can't help with challenging interpersonal situations, such as divorce or a partner or spouse leaving. And the worst situation has been seeing a patient go into a nursing home when they couldn't be looked after by their family any longer. I just couldn't do anything to help and that was horrible.

But as MS nurses, there are so many more things we can do now to assist a patient build strong and stable mental health. Back when I started, even trying to monitor such treacherous tendencies as suicide was very difficult. We just didn't have the skills or the resources to help in that way. These days we have a wealth of information and far better research that aids us in picking up the clues and hints to people's cognitive deficits and also emerging or lingering mental health issues. And it's also because we inherently believe that people can live a much better life after a diagnosis of MS.

At the Center, we would have team meetings every week to talk about these problems and just try and unload amongst each other. It was an opportunity for us to talk about our feelings, the feelings in general of the work we do and to work between each other to develop care strategies not only for ourselves but also our patients. I think team meetings in a clinical environment are just so vital and also for me personally, I like to ensure I always have a quiet place that is 'MS Free.' That spot for me is with my family, or whilst reading, listening to music or even just taking a hot bath. There are just things you've got to do to take care of yourself so as you can take care of others.

And I believe this is true even for those living with MS. You have to have a 'MS Free Zone' in your life. It should be a place that MS doesn't belong. Ros Kalb talked about that years ago and I've always subscribed to the notion. A MS Free Zone is vital for the patient, for the family and for the health care team because you simply can't live and breathe multiple sclerosis 24 hours a day, seven days a week. You'll go bonkers otherwise!

Rosalind C Kalb, a clinical psychologist and also the vice president of the Professional Resource Center at the National MS Society in the USA, wrote the 2007 book 'Multiple Sclerosis: The Questions You Have-The Answers You Need.'

In the book, she talks about the practice, and indeed survival technique, of establishing a MS Free Zone.

She explains that for someone living with MS, if the disease course has forced them to give up one or another activity that has been important in their life, try to experiment with other activities or pursuits that may turn out to be equally satisfying. Most importantly, she coaches, 'look for that aspect of yourself that MS is unable to touch.' For one person, it may be their sense of humour, for another their religious beliefs and for yet another, their love of music. Kalb encourages that by identifying this MS Free Zone within yourself, you can retain a sense of who you are, even in the face of stressful changes. The MS Free Zone can also be an important source of emotional energy, a place within yourself that you can go to refuel when the challenges of everyday life leave you feeling drained or overwhelmed. Breaking the illness down into individual challenges is a way of trying to 'win the war;' it provides a sense that the patient and even their family are managing the MS, rather than the other way around.

And I guess that identification of hope and joy even amongst the fear of living with an uncertain illness is key for me.

Many people have actually written about the concept of hope and how it applies to nursing. And I've adapted the hope model and would always tell my patients to never lose hope. That single point alone is very important and empowering. Hope for a cure, hope for the treatment, hope for a clinician that cares. There just needs to be hope ingrained with all the positive things that you do, no matter whether you're a nurse or a person living with MS or have a loved one with MS.

And hope alone is no good unless you're prepared to be proactive in your own health. And also keep in mind that people find hope in a lot of different ways.

Throughout the course of my career I've met many amazing people in the field of MS, people with a lot of talent and dedication but it was actually one of my patients who inspired me early in my career and I've never forgotten her.

I met this particular woman back in 1978. Her name was Helen, but she didn't like to be called by that, she insisted I call her Lee.

She was 29 years old and had a wonderful career ahead of her when she was diagnosed with MS. When I met her, I was working in public health and I'd been assigned to go and see her to treat an extremely bad bed sore. This thing was the size of a cantaloupe and ran very deep. She wanted to go to a rehab facility that was close by. It was the only facility existing then (and remains the only facility that was ever available) to specifically rehabilitate people with MS. Anyway, she was determined to walk again and the facility wouldn't take her back for rehab until that bedsore was healed. So every day I went back to see her and every weekend I'd be reading about new research and ways to treat bed sores. I would work every single day – seven days a week – to treat that wound. We eventually closed the wound and she said 'Right. Now I can go and walk again.' I thought to myself – very cynically – 'sure thing….'

Well let me tell you what happened! She went to this rehab facility and they got her into leg braces and she did walk again! Her determination gave me the inspiration to stay in MS. Even when I transitioned from public health and went back to school to get my advanced degree I went to see her to tell her how influenced I was by her determination and spirit. Coincidentally, many years later I ordered a car service to get to the airport and the driver said 'Oh! You're June Halper?'

'Well, yes…' I replied.

He then went on to tell me he was Helen's brother and that she always talked about me and that bond we had. Helen very much inspired me with her prevailing spirit of hope and determination. She just never gave up.

I don't think I could capture and convey four decades of nursing into one small sound bite of advice, but I do believe that among the many responsibilities of the MS nurse, perhaps the most important is to help patients devise, learn, and implement self-care strategies to improve their wellness and quality of life. And I would similarly apply this statement to nurses assisting nurses.

The caregiver role takes many forms and could be defined as somebody professional, such as a nurse, a physician, a rehab specialist, mental health expert but also the family or friends of the person with MS. The caregiving model in MS is extremely important, because it's a disease that lasts a lifetime and trying to tackle this by yourself is a lonely job. So, everyone needs someone who understands what you've been through.

And it's a two-way street. People with MS need the support from a variety of people and resources to 'win the war,' but so too do the nurses. There may have only been a handful of MS nurses when I started out, but what a wonderous thing we've created amongst our global peers today to be able to easily connect with others that intimately understand our feelings and can quell that fear of isolation or the feeling of uncertainty, and similarly share the triumph of a win. Just remember.....everyone needs their A team!

My hopes for the future treatment and management of MS:

• I hope that someone, someday will figure out what causes or triggers MS. Just think then about how we might be able to create targeted treatments if we knew more about the cause... Diagnosis would very likely be a faster process and even prevention might be possible.

• And whilst talking about causes, I think there's a lot of optimism around studying the genetics of MS so that we can personalise the treatments. I look at the great things that scientists are doing within the field of cancer research and genetics and the possibility of targeting gene therapies for the treatment of MS is exciting to me.

• The greatest advance in the treatment of MS I've seen over the course of my career has been the emergence of the MS nurse. This definite shift to having the advanced practice nurse so intrinsically involved in the patient's treatment protocol is incredibly significant. It's a positive allocation of resources, alleviating the pressure from the neurologist yet still providing the person living with MS much readier access to an integral specialist.

My advice for nurses beginning their career:

• Those nurses starting out need to become highly educated; they need to commit to continual education. I see a wave where MS is being seen as only a DMT disease. A lot of nurses are coming into MS believing the only thing they need to do is get the patient onto a disease modifying therapy. That is absolutely not the case. You have to address the total patient and you've got to learn all about MS. Then when you're meeting with your patient, you've got to discover the primary area of concern in that person's life and address it first. With a great deal of patients, they are experiencing challenges in their lives that have everything to do with MS but no DMT will ever fix it – let alone the patients who aren't prescribed DMTs.

• Quite simply, what matters most to the patient should matter most to you. Generally what matters most to the patient is something that a symptom or the disease course is compromising and causing the patient's life to go down the tubes.

• I once met a guy from Merck Pharmaceutical who confided in me one of his motivating factors to work in health care. He said to me 'over the year, the one thing I've always kept in mind is not what I'm trying to accomplish but I have to remember that the patient is waiting.' So no matter whether we consider ourselves the A team at the centre or whatever other label we give ourselves as health care providers, we have to keep reminding ourselves why we're in the business. We're in this to take care of people with MS. And what matters most to them should matter most to me.

• The other piece of advice I'd give to a nurse starting out is to listen. Find your colleagues and listen to them and draw advice and inspiration from them. Likewise, really listen to your patients and fully understand what their needs are. Perhaps what they want to learn about is not actually what you want to teach them. Always be open to new ideas and to learning and to growth; don't allow yourself to get stuck in the same old rut. Try to learn every day!

JOELLE MASSOUH
Beirut, Lebanon

"People often wonder about the differences I might contend with each day in Beirut, but I think no matter where you are in the world, living with and working in MS brings its own set of idiosyncrasies but also enormous commonalities."

No matter what image you have in your mind of Beirut, it's a very close-knit community. The media doesn't always paint a great picture of my home town, but I feel rooted in this city and also this setting. Maybe it's because I was actually born in the same hospital that I now work. I walk to work every day and walked to university and my classes before that. So as much as we think of Beirut as being a big chaotic city, I have very much been able to find my own feeling of community here; for me, it's really just like a small town! People get to know each other and naturally, us Lebanese like to share a lot of 'information' amongst one another, so we form close bonds!

My career in MS nursing is shorter compared to many of my foreign colleagues, mainly due to the fact that our MS centre in Lebanon was only established a short time ago.

I graduated from the American University of Beirut (AUB)

a little over ten years ago with a Bachelor of Science in nursing and immediately started working in a specialty medical-surgical in-patient unit that serviced a large concentration of oncology cases. And whilst the facility also catered to neurological conditions, for my first few years of nursing I spent most of my time with oncology patients, looking after a range of their needs, administering chemotherapy and also attending to palliative care.

The American University is the largest university in Lebanon and has been ranked as the number one educational institution in the region. It is also rich in history. The story of our medical center – the American University of Beirut Medical Centre (AUBMC) – began 145 years ago in a small rented building in Zokak El-Blat in Beirut. It was originally home to the first classes of the School of Medicine, which was established by the Syrian Protestant College, and later became known as AUB. It became evident, and quite quickly, that the School of Medicine would need to expand to meet the needs and demands of our region. Subsequently, my school of nursing, the first of its kind in the Middle East, was founded in 1905.

Only four years into my own nursing career, an opportunity presented itself for me to be part of a multiple sclerosis centre that was to be established as part of the AUBMC 2020 Vision Plan to develop more centres of excellence in the country.

Essentially, the AUBMC 2020 Vision Plan predicated that the AUB should build on its strong foundations in medical education and health care. In addition to improving facilities and capacity, the AUBMC 2020 Vision set out to establish centres of excellence that would provide new medical options for the treatment of illnesses endemic in the Arab world. The plan also allowed for expansion and access to the quality of care that families in Lebanon have depended on for generations.

The strategy really was incredibly exciting. Launched in 2010, the AUBMC 2020 Vision was an ambitious and comprehensive initiative that affirmed AUBMC's position as the leading medical centre and healthcare institution in the region. The strategy transformed medical education, research and practice, and most importantly, national medical care, creating new levels of excellence. The initiative established several major new medical facilities – both clinical and academic – and also established clinical and research centres of excellence. There was heavy investment in state-of-the-art equipment, and a focus on recruiting talented physicians and nurses, and building regional and international partnerships.

I interviewed for this new role with Dr. Samia Khoury, who was to be the director of the MS centre being established in Beirut. I was excited to meet Dr. Khoury; she was previously the co-director of a centre in Harvard, USA called the Partners Multiple Sclerosis Center.

This particular centre, located at Brigham and Women's Hospital (BWH) in Boston, is world renowned for providing the most advanced multiple sclerosis treatment options for patients with MS, and it is bolstered by a clinical research program that is leading the way in the latest multiple sclerosis discoveries. Since its creation in 1999, the Center, led by Howard L. Weiner, MD, has been at the forefront of MS patient care and research, including the landmark Comprehensive Longitudinal Investigation of Multiple Sclerosis at BWH (CLIMB) study that has provided many insights into genetics, immunology, imaging and treatment of multiple sclerosis.

Dr. Khoury left the Brigham to come back to Lebanon and open the MS centre at the AUBMC. She is recognised as a world leader in MS, having trained many investigators who are now active leaders in MS and Immunology research. She has published over 200 scholarly articles, reviews, and book chapters. Moreover, she led the first National Multiple Sclerosis awareness campaign in Lebanon in collaboration with the Ministry of Public Health for the year 2013. To say I was intrigued was an understatement. As a feminist, I was especially proud that a woman would lead this centre in my country.

During those first four years in nursing I had made it a habit to read about the work of other specialty nurses and also speak with nurses who had chosen to specialise. I knew that specialising in a field was a way I could make a big difference. Multiple sclerosis really intrigued me; I had already met a few MS patients whilst working at the in-patient ward when I would assist with the infusions of steroids and some of the DMTs. I saw that MS was a disease of young people, particularly women, and that adjusting to a lifelong disease was challenging. I wanted to be part of the support team that helped them.

I was successfully appointed to one of the two nursing positions available at the new MS centre, and in the eight short but fast-paced years since we began, the centre has grown exponentially. We started with one patient per week and now we have close to two thousand patients overall. The majority of the patients living with MS in Lebanon will be treated at our centre.

It's difficult to determine how many people are living with MS in Lebanon. No official census has been undertaken since 1932 due to the sensitive balance between the country's religious groups, but it's been estimated by a variety of organisations that the country has a population of approximately six million. Of this total population, some five million are Lebanese nationals, with a belief that there is a further one million to 1.5 million people from Syria, Palestine or Iraq living in Lebanon as either refugees or alyssum seekers. Between a lack of census information – and with a fluctuating influx of refugees into Lebanon – accounting for both population and health statistics of any cohort is nearly impossible.

Whilst we have some statistics from the Ministry of Health around the number of people taking a MS medication, we also recognise that there are many people diagnosed with MS who don't, or can't, take a medication, so once again our figures remain a bit unknown. Because our health system in Lebanon doesn't provide for unique patient identification numbers, as it does in other countries, we also can't fully determine if there's a replication of patient figures between different hospitals in Lebanon, adding more ambiguity.

We have certainly started a registry at our MS centre, but it just takes time to build historical data and obviously, an updated national census would aid us.

So up until the establishment of the MS Centre in 2011, I had only seen a few MS patients for infusions. Their own diagnosis was so new and at that time, I didn't have much more than a very generalised knowledge about MS. It wasn't until I started at the MS centre that my real on-the-job training started!

We began the Center with two MS specialists. The first was our director Dr. Khoury and the other was a neurologist, Dr. Bassem Yamout, who had a background in MS from a smaller centre where he'd also been involved in some research projects. Our managing director was a nurse who'd completed some training in MS at The Brigham prior to our clinic opening and the team was rounded out with a specialist MS pharmacist who had also been recruited from another clinic. We were only a small group and our practical training was intense. I supplemented my own on-the-job training with a lot of self-learning. I was constantly reading about MS and best-practice principals and the latest research into the disease. Pretty much anything I could get my hands onto! I eventually started studying for my master's degree in nursing a few years back so I could focus on neurology and multiple sclerosis, which also assisted enormously.

I came across the International Organization for MS Nurses (IOMSN) during the extensive amount of time I spent on the web reading about MS. Right away I was really intrigued because I have a tremendous passion for my career and I remember feeling so proud at the discovery of the organisation. Imagine finding a group of other nurses who shared that passion and had been working in the field for a long time!

Going to my first annual conference for the Consortium of Multiple Sclerosis Centers (CMSC) in 2014 was a turning point in my career. Prior to the conference, I had looked into the prospect of sitting the certification exam to become a MS Specialist Nurse; I knew I didn't have as many years' experience as other nurses in the field but I had my heart set on becoming a specialist in MS. The certification has the reputation of being quite onerous and intense and I knew I was in for a great deal of study. On top of this, we had no established testing facilities in Lebanon for me to sit the exam – I daresay because no one in my country had taken the exam before – but I was able to work with the IOMSN and the Multiple Sclerosis Nurses International Certification Board to organise a formal testing process at the university in Beirut.

I successfully sat the exam and gained my certification and it was an immediate confidence boost! The credentials are well-recognised and held in high esteem and it was also a great experience to be attending my first CMSC conference as an already-credentialed MS Specialist Nurse. And conversely, it was very interesting for my western colleagues to meet someone from a very different country to their own! We swapped some wonderful stories and I met some inspiring nurses with decades of experience. Knowing I had a whole professional community who could support me was very comforting, particularly given we were only newly-established in my country.

I still continue to be grateful for the access to a group of people who have a wealth of clinical knowledge and personal insights from a wide variety of patients; just knowing I can quickly connect with other people who 'get it.' It's an enriching experience.

***

I found it equally exciting and scary to be at the coalface of a brand-new initiative in Lebanon. Something that hadn't been seen in our country before now. The Nehme and Therese Tohme Multiple Sclerosis Center was designed to function as a dedicated clinic for MS patients, with both in-patient and out-patient facilities, and also a treatment infusion centre.

For the first few weeks after opening the clinic in 2011, we only had one patient a week. I remember how excited we were about that first patient! It probably sounds a bit strange, but my nursing colleague and myself were so giddy with excitement that we fought over who would see the patient!

It was a bit slow going initially, until the centre started to become recognised by other specialists and also the MS community itself. We were additionally getting a bit of push back from some neurologists who wanted to keep patients under their own care. Perhaps in those early days they didn't understand the need for a comprehensive treatment centre or they simply didn't know enough about the MS Centre itself?

So our centre launched an awareness campaign in conjunction with the Ministry of Health and from that point forward, we started to see more referrals from neurologists and enquiries from people living with MS. Concurrent to that, interest in MS in general was growing. We were increasing our patient numbers week by week and recently had to expand our facilities to accommodate extra patient rooms and also recruit a third nurse to assist us clinically. Our research team had been growing quite consistently since we started but our clinical team has only just been able to catch up to our needs. We would be considered a small centre by global standards, but it's certainly not small for Lebanon.

We now see up to sixty patients a week across both the clinic and for infusions. We basically increased sixty-fold in six years! And we still continue to receive new patient referrals every week. It has been overwhelming because we want to cater to everyone in the best way possible, however the increase has been quite steep to manage, but no matter, I still find it such a rewarding role.

During the awareness campaign, we had a lot of people presenting to the clinic who didn't really fit the criteria of having MS. They may have been experiencing intermittent symptoms or some numbness or loss of sensation, however we mostly knew that what a person was experiencing was definitely not MS. But because there was just so much more information for the general public to now read about the disease, we were having so much more enquiry. Certainly, there were instances where people were scared about the small things that might be slightly similar to a MS symptom and we even saw quite a few people confusing amyotrophic lateral sclerosis (ALS) and multiple sclerosis (MS). We had to find a way to regulate the people who had seen the national awareness campaign and became convinced that they had MS; we had to develop a basic screening process for our clinic assistant, which included asking if the person had obtained an MRI or been referred to the centre specifically by a family doctor.

At the clinic, we don't actually consult with anyone who has had no prior indication of MS. If they haven't had an MRI or been referred directly by a family doctor or neurologist, we'll ask that they take a step back and seek some initial clarity via those health care providers.

Lebanon is a small country where everyone knows everyone and that trickles down to everyone knowing a doctor. So if someone is experiencing symptoms that are suggestive of MS, and they've undergone a brain MRI that has revealed suspicious lesions and then been referred to the Center, we'll nearly always have the doctor ringing on behalf of their patient and trying to get them seen earlier. We'll always do our best to see the patient extremely quickly so as we don't lose the opportunity to do our own extensive MRI exams and make a conclusive diagnosis.

Some seven or eight years down the track from our original awareness campaign we can see that it has worked because people are generally more aware of what MS is and is not. Combined with far better and faster diagnostic processes and the outcome is that we have become quite adept at managing and supporting our growing patient enquiry and load. It's been quite intriguing to see the change, especially when you factor in we started from nowhere!

***

*Collaboration is our key to working through
the diagnostic process*

Without doubt, one of the first questions people want to know, is if what they are feeling is MS or not? They may be referred to the centre only knowing that their MRI has noted 'demyleanating lesions' or 'suspicious of MS.' So a definitive diagnosis is a priority for them. And like anywhere around the world, some of these diagnoses are challenging because the person in front of us may not precisely fit the McDonald criteria. They might be CIS or RIS and we'll have to take quite a bit of time explaining the difference between the two and what it may mean for them in terms of the disease course and monitoring.

Magnetic resonance imaging has improved the diagnosis and evaluation of disease activity in MS, and its widespread use has contributed to creating the concept of 'radiologically isolated syndrome' (RIS) to describe patients without symptoms of MS whose MRI findings suggest they might be at risk of future demyelinating events. Indeed, using the revised McDonald criteria now allows some patients who would have been diagnosed with 'clinically isolated syndrome' (CIS) in the era of the Poser criteria to be diagnosed as having MS before a second episode.

Of course, the other big questions that frequently arise are whether they can continue working or studying, right through to whether they'll be able to get married and have children.

That first visit might be a bit overwhelming for someone newly diagnosed so we simply try to provide support. I'll generally suggest more frequent visits to the clinic to navigate the early days so as we can gradually provide information and make plans rather than overloading the patient and their family. If the patient has been prescribed intravenous methylprednisolone steroids to stem that first exacerbation, it actually gives our team an opportunity to see them every day for a few days, gently providing a bit of new information on each visit and also answering their questions as they process more and more.

Developing our systems from the ground up has meant we've been able to take bits and pieces of processes from clinics globally to create our own work flow. A new patient visiting the MS Center will begin with a clinic assistant who fills in the necessary administrative documentation. After this, the patient will be handed off to a nurse's aide who will prep the patient for the MS team's consultation. We ensure that the interactions between our entire MS medical team and the patient all happen in the same meeting area. We don't want our patient and their family to be shuffled amongst various hospital rooms.

This initial patient consultation with the team will begin with the MS nurse obtaining a detailed medical history and then if the suspicion of MS is quite high, we'll perform the MSFC test.

According to the National MS Society in the United States, The Multiple Sclerosis Functional Composite (MSFC) is a three-part, standardised, quantitative assessment instrument for use in clinical studies, (particularly clinical trials) of MS. It was developed by a special Task Force on Clinical Outcomes Assessment that had been appointed by the National Multiple Sclerosis Society's Advisory Committee on Clinical Trials of New Agents in MS. It was the consensus of the task force that important clinical dimensions not emphasised in existing rating scales should be measured. Measures of cognition are an example of this.

The MSFC was designed to fulfil three criteria:

1. It should be multidimensional to reflect the varied clinical expression of MS across both the patient and over time.

2. The dimensions should change relatively independently over time.

3. One component should be a measure of cognitive function.

The three components of the MSFC measure leg function/ ambulation, arm/hand function, and cognitive function.

The MS nurse will then present the patient's information to the entire team, which may include the neurological and clinical research fellows – along with our core team of the neurologists, other MS nurses and the MS pharmacist. In addition to the MS nurse's presentation, we'll also assess any other materials we have available, such as MRI's and lumbar puncture test results. After this, the neurologist will perform an expanded disability status scale (EDSS) and will also have a chance to discuss the impression and the results privately with the patient. At this point – and if the patient is comfortable with everything – they may ask the family to join the team for the remainder of the process.

While I was completing my master's degree I was required to do a residency at another MS centre for nearly two months. With the assistance of Dr. Khoury, I chose to undertake that residency at Partners Multiple Sclerosis Center at Brigham and Women's Hospital in Boston because there was no other multidisciplinary MS centre in the Middle East region.

My residency was incredibly interesting. The Partners MS Center is a huge facility with a lot of providers but only one clinical MS nurse. I learned that in their system, the MS nurse worked in isolation with the patient, rather than being part of the patient's round-table care team. Instead they utilise nurse practitioners (NPs), which in itself was fascinating for me as we don't have such a role in Lebanon; as MS nurses we don't have prescriptive or diagnostic authority. I had met many nurse practitioners before but working closely with the NPs was extremely intriguing to see the difference in their consultations with patients compared to ours at the clinic in Lebanon. Even the way the NPs interacted with their patients compared to how the neurologists would consult with the same patient was fascinating. I could feel the NPs approach was very wholesome and holistic.

I admire the comprehensive and collaborative approach we have fostered at our centre in Beirut. As the centre becomes busier, it is becoming more difficult for the nurse to remain with the patient for the entire round-table process, but we're there for it as much as possible and I'm hopeful that as our nursing resources increase we can be there from start to finish.

From the inception of the Center's development, we have been able to work in a small team to walk our patient through a comprehensive intake process. Perhaps in the very beginning there was a small amount of opposition to the MS nurse being the primary point of contact in the centre. I think it may have been difficult, not just for other neurologists to grasp and accept, but even the patients. In our paternalistic culture, patients will hold a doctor's opinion in greater esteem than a nurse's. In those early days we would be questioned by the patients and their families as to why they weren't being seen by a doctor first? And that was initially difficult because they clearly didn't understand our role in the centre and just how much of a support we would become to them on this journey. All we could do was to keep working diligently to change the mentality.

And I do believe the change of mentality has come full circle, because now, if a patient doesn't see you when they visit the clinic, they will ask for you specifically. My own role as the MS nurse in our clinic means that I'm a primary contact in their clinical experience. Other nurses, research fellows and clinical assistants have come and gone, but I'm still there!

The clinic has only been going eight years, but for some patients, I've been alongside them as they've experienced major milestones in life, such as graduating university, getting married or having children.

Ensuring that I gain the trust and confidence of the patient from the beginning is highly important. In Lebanon, our role as out-patient nurses is not seen as being as experienced or possessing the comprehensive range of skills as other nurses, yet I believe the specialisation I've chosen provides me far greater scope than many others.

People often wonder about the differences I might contend with each day in Beirut, compared to say Chicago or London or Sydney? But I think no matter where you are in the world, living with and working in MS brings its own set of idiosyncrasies – depending on the cultural and geographical implications – but also enormous commonalities.

The extended family unit is important to the Lebanese people, as it provides a high level of support and even functions as a type of social security system. And naturally, within this support structure, the role of the mother is supremely authoritative, especially in the level of influence she is able to wield over her children. I've learned to craft that healthy balance where I can honour the family's urge to be intimately involved in every decision whilst still maintaining a patient's privacy. This is no easy feat when dealing with overly-protective mums – although that may be a phenomenon that occurs worldwide! I often get mothers asking me to tell their sons that they should stop smoking the hookah pipes. I have many situations where I have to weigh up whether I'm sounding like I'm collaborating with their mother or actually just sounding like their MS nurse!

I have also seen some pressure on my female patients, that come from more conservative families or towns, with regards to genetics and family planning. This is particularly obvious if the patient is yet to conceive a boy; I think sometimes the family would rather see their daughter or wife come off the MS medication and instead try to conceive a son. But if my patient has a particularly active disease course or is progressing, my preference is for them to remain on treatment. It can be a challenging situation to navigate in our culture.

MS can present as a reasonably silent or invisible disease in a lot of people, and I often find I need to guide a patient's family, friends and work or study colleagues to be somewhat empathetic. Those 'invisible' symptoms are very real and require the support – or at the very least the belief that they exist – from everyone.

And whilst I respect and admire the power of the family unit, I personally draw the line at giving any information to my patient's family members without their consent. The role of the family is so strong in our culture and I know it must be difficult for some doctors to make that distinction, but for me, the patient is my primary concern.

I'm sure I experience many of the same frustrations in nursing and caring for my patients as my colleagues around the world. I know from talking with other MS nurses that we all feel the pain when we can't do enough for a patient.

For me, this is especially true in the situations where I'm working with a patient who is quite progressed in their disease course and showing signs of severe disability; I wish I could do more. And in the same vein, I feel so deeply for those patients whose symptoms are just not improving despite the many interventions we've instituted. I just feel like my hands are tied and it does upset me. I feel like I'm trying my best but the limitations that I can't overcome are just so frustrating. And these limitations are two-fold; it could be that the disease is progressing in a way that is difficult for us to intervene but at other times it might be that we just don't have access to a treatment or standard of care that is effective.

And another challenge I often face is helping my patients transfer their care to other countries. It happens quite a bit in Lebanon as people frequently travel for work, education or family commitments. Obviously not all counties have the same treatment guidelines and different clinics will also have their own way of doing things. One particular patient of mine wasn't given access to her normal medication when she moved to Europe. Consequently, she was put onto another disease modifying therapy (DMT) and suffered terribly from adverse side effects. She was constantly in contact with us and asking for advice, but it was so difficult to support this patient; I just wanted to put her back on her regular treatment but my hands were tied; I knew the other clinic was well within their rights to treat their patient the way they thought they needed to.

And then of course, in Lebanon, we're dealing with a burgeoning refugee population from Syria, Palestine and right through to patients visiting from Iraq. In any given week, around twenty percent of the people I see may be living as a refugee. There are so many cultural differences we need to take into consideration with these patients and of top of that, we experience a lot of challenges in arranging follow up consultations or providing them with ongoing access to care. Our Ministry for Health can only provide medications for Lebanese nationals, which is naturally challenging for us when we're treating people with MS.

In Lebanon, if a person with MS is working, the National Social Security Fund (NSSF) will cover a share of the various aspects of treatment, such as medications, hospitalisation, MRIs and so on. The proportion covered is roughly eighty to ninety percent of the care. In the case where a Lebanese citizen is not working and does not have access to the NSSF, they still qualify to have chronic medications dispensed via a special Ministry of Health programme, however, this programme would cover the medications only, leaving the consultations, hospitalisation and anything else as the financial responsibility of the patient. Private health insurance programmes may cover some of the short fall in those instances, but generally the insurance still falls far short.

Which is where our 'Friends of MS Fund' comes in. The fund – raised purely through the charity of others – will help tremendously in filling that financial gap.

In the case of the refugees, we rely on wealthy benefactors and the philanthropy of business people from countries such as Syria to help support our care fund.

With the refugee patients I see, it's not only the disease course of multiple sclerosis they are dealing with. Living in those camps is tough and accessing the other types of health care they need for health issues other than MS can be difficult. And at our MS clinic, we can't help them with everything, so as a nurse, I find that quite emotionally difficult. Sometimes they don't even have the money to get a ride from their camp to the clinic. It's really tough when we just can't do enough.

***

Keeping the bigger picture in mind

It would be easy to get lost in the small details of the very broad range of situations we have to face every day.

In fact, the diversity of responsibilities I have to handle on a daily basis could certainly become overwhelming. If I have a lot of administrative tasks to take care of, I'll often think to myself I could be better using that time to talk with my patients, rather than doing paperwork or spending far too long on the phone sorting out non-clinical issues. I really enjoy working with my patients and I'd rather dedicate my time and expertise there. And certainly on those heavy administrative days, I might leave the clinic feeling as if the whole point of the day has been missed. I know some of those administrative details may be helping someone in the end, but my passion simply lies in the direct patient interaction. And I guess that's where learning to structure your day appropriately is hugely beneficial. Looking at your day so as you can give the best of your time to the things that really matter to you.

And for me, it's not just thinking about the day ahead, but I also try to make sure the bigger picture of what I wish to achieve in my career is being factored in. And this is where continuing my education, keeping abreast of research and voraciously reading scholarly articles comes in. But also, reading and listening to the stories of MS patients shapes my view of what I'd like to achieve in my career as a MS nurse.

Being the first certified MS specialist nurse in the country has provided many opportunities for me to travel to regional and international conferences to share my experiences and importantly, learn from others. These conferences are for both patients and also other medical professionals and the experiences have helped me grow my own community of MS nurses and colleagues.

Whilst broadening our nursing community is tremendously important and obviously beneficial in how we care for those with MS, it has also helped me become better at my own job because to be able to teach other people, you have to keep learning every day as well.

And conversely, attending a great variety of conferences all around the world has allowed me to learn from all my own role models. These wonderful people and experiences allow me to continue nurturing something I'm passionate about and in turn, I'm able to give back to that same community as the middle-eastern delegate on the MS Nurses International Certification Board. Being invited to fill that role, but also just continually networking with other nurses in this specialised field around the world, has been an enormous boost to my confidence and of course my ability. All these things just make my heart grow!

All the support I get from my international colleagues is very important. I didn't have any significant MS role models in Lebanon because essentially, this specialised field didn't exist before the Center was founded. I was learning from neurologists – and that was rewarding – but learning from other nurses specifically is very important because you have to be able to confide in and learn from other people that you can find a common ground with.

At a recent middle east regional MS nurses conference, I was talking to a colleague I greatly admire, Therese Burke. I was explaining the challenges I was facing in bringing together our community of nurses within that region, due to the vast distances, lack of infrastructure and also language barriers. Therese was able to give me tremendous hope and great advice that the challenges I was facing certainly weren't insurmountable.

Whilst we might consider countries such as Australia, America and even the United Kingdom as being quite developed, they still face very similar challenges as we do in the middle east in having to overcome problems in treating patients in remote areas and also managing with limited resources. She made me believe that anything was possible. It might take time and a lot of passion, but it was possible to create a strong community of MS nurses.

It also requires having people in leadership positions believe in you. Dr. Bassem Yamout, president of the Middle East North Africa Committee for Treatment and Research in MS (MENACTRIMS) and a mentor I learn from daily, did just that. He supported me in growing a community of MENA region MS nurses through my position as the MENACTRIMS Nursing Program Coordinator, where I organise a full day parallel nursing session at the annual MENACTRIMS congress.

***

MS will 'fit' into their life. It won't 'become' their life.

I remember when I was first starting out and before I was able to gain a worldlier view of MS care and how patients live with this disease, it was definitely more difficult for me to help my patients see a big picture.

But with time comes experience and over time I saw more and more people living really well – in fact doing amazing things – whilst living with MS. It was then that I was able to convince my own patients that life does go on. That those difficult adjustment times in the first few years may seem impossible, but they will get through it.

I see that many patients initially develop a mindset after their diagnosis that if anything bad that could possibly happen, it will surely happen to them. And similarly, any small ailment or health anomaly is immediately attributed to MS, which we know is not always the case. And I absolutely understand that fear. All of a sudden, their world view narrows to focus only on their own life as they try to survive those early days. But now that I have many more years of specialist MS nursing under my belt, I can confidently explain to them that what they are feeling is actually quite normal and so many other people with MS feel the same way. I'm not aiming to invalidate their fears, but more to re-assure them that they are not alone. For those patients that are open to it, I try to match them with another person living with MS who is similar in their character and stage of life and perhaps experiencing similar types of symptoms. I find that those conversations between two people living with MS can be helpful in solidifying the messages or resources I can provide.

I've personally weathered periods of depression in my life and going through this experience – and managing it – has definitely helped me in assisting my patients. I know I can share and understand this particular experience with them, even if I can't fully put myself in their shoes when it comes to other MS symptoms. I don't shy away from difficult conversations such as suicidal ideations; I prefer to tackle them head on. There's a popular page on Facebook called 'Humans of New York' that shares portraits and powerful stories from New Yorkers, and there's an especially powerful quote from a depressed psychiatrist that resonates so much with me: "When I'm ready to get my license, there will be a question on the application that says: Have you ever had a mental illness that impaired your ability to treat patients? I'm going to answer no. Because being a patient has been a revelatory experience. It's taught me how difficult it can be to verbalize what you're feeling. And it's taught me the power of denial, even for someone who studies the symptoms. When I began the medication, it was like a veil had been lifted from my eyes. So much of what I know about depression, I learned by getting through it."

And I also know my capacity and perspective to deal with tough situations in MS nursing has been shaped by my previous role working in oncology. Back then, the days were long because I didn't want to miss talking to patients who really needed support during treatments and I also wanted to be sure my charting was as comprehensive as possible. I was just starting out in my nursing career, and I was trying to develop good habits early. And there were times these long days took a toll on my mental health, as did loosing so many patients to a disease like cancer that has such a high mortality rate in my country. But it was important to me to make their end-of-life experience as peaceful as possible. It was definitely taxing emotionally, but the role I had to play in their transition was something I knew I had to do. I am eternally grateful for all those patients who have allowed me into their lives before they passed on.

Playing a major role in a patient's care is inherent in me and consequently, the move into MS nursing was intuitive after my experience in oncology. Becoming a surgical nurse or a trauma nurse was not personally appealing. I knew I wanted to work with people who were dealing with a chronic condition but I definitely didn't want to work in providing palliative care any longer. I needed to head towards something a bit more hopeful.

And the longer I work in MS, I realise that those experiences gained from providing end-of-life comfort are quite transferable in helping people with MS grieve a previous way of life. My patients may be losing function, losing something they could once do but no longer can, losing support of family or friends. There's a lot of loss in MS and working with oncology patients definitely prepared me better for this. I know I can talk very candidly and with expertise to my patients that MS is not a disease they will die from and that while they are alive, there's still a lot of things we can do and a lot of ways we can help them live the fullest life possible. It can be particularly challenging for those patients facing difficult losses – at any time throughout their disease course – because at that point, the loss can be quite consuming: It can be their sole focus. So working alongside those people to find a level of acceptance and also perspective and hope can be interesting.

I find the topic of resilience very fascinating. In fact, it's the topic I tackled in my master's research; I wanted to explore why people with a severe disability may be able to better adjust to the 'new way of life' than those people with less challenges? I am looking into the association of anxiety, depression, personality type, and social support with resilience. Analysing the data is quite interesting especially given the current revolution in Lebanon and its effect on people's psyche and subsequently their MS. My hope is to be able to work on future interventions that can help people with MS bounce back and develop what is known as post-traumatic growth. A poignant, personal favourite quote by Mahmoud Darwish translates to "And I say to myself: a moon will rise from my darkness."

One of the most important things I want those newly diagnosed with MS to know is that MS will 'fit' into their life. It won't 'become' their life. They will learn over time to be able to just get on with their life and not be defined by it.

I also want new nurses to understand how empowering it is to be part of the process in helping our patients manage MS. In fact, the role of the MS nurse is integral within our patient's lives. We don't just fit IVs and write charts. We get the opportunity to really talk with our patients in more depth and gain a deeper understanding of their daily challenges (and wins!) of living with MS. We do have the opportunity to gain more than just the routine snapshot of their life.

This is a vocation that will absolutely shape you and that process for growth and learning is very important for nurses. Being able to spend time with patients provides a lasting imprint on your personality and psyche for ever. I've had patients who have left a lasting impression on my life and these experiences help us to help the next person. Over the last few years I've trained a lot of colleagues in our centre and I know it can all be a bit overwhelming in the beginning, particularly if they haven't worked closely with disability before coming into our field. And it can also be confronting at times, but I try to help them see the big picture with MS; to understand that their role in helping patients better adjust to life is so greatly rewarding and that people with MS can live an incredibly full life.

Author's Note:

Only months after this interview, Joelle was the inaugural recipient of the International MS Nursing Leadership Award. This award was established to honor the memory of Nicola "Nicki" Ward-Abel who embodied the best in MS Nursing. She was an expert clinician, leader, mentor, and role model. The award acknowledges those qualities in MS nurses who practice throughout the world.

My hopes for the future treatment and management of MS:

•   One of the greatest reasons for hope comes in seeing the increased availability of more treatment options, particularly transitioning solely from injectable treatments to now having a range of orals, infusions and treatments that are just easier to tailor to a patient's own disease course and symptoms. Compliance with treatment is far better because of the variety of options we now have. Patients are far more likely to stay on a treatment that is easier to manage and that actually works for them. And because we have the full range of options available in Lebanon, the patients are more involved in the decision-making process when choosing a treatment, so are more accepting of the risk that these treatments involve.

•   Being able to tell my patients that in just a decade we have gone from having only few injectable treatments to being able to offer a dozen-plus treatments – including the first approved DMT for progressive MS – is pretty remarkable. And on top of that, to re-assure them of the headway being made into the research of repair and remyelination is really hopeful. In my mind, these are milestone achievements.

•   I know this sounds like a really bizarre thing to say, but I tell my patients that if ever there was a time to have MS (not that you'd ever choose to!) now would be the time. We are living in an era of massive advances and possibilities for how we manage the disease, and this was not the case only ten to fifteen year ago.

•   I also don't talk to my patients only in terms of 'finding a cure.' That's a lot of pressure and hope for anyone to hold and I think there are going to be so many ways in which we tackle this disease in the future.

My advice for nurses beginning their career:

•   When I was working as an in-patient nurse, I truly believed I had the most opportunity to really help (and even save) my patients. The work was immediate and often critical. But since becoming an MS nurse in an out-patient clinic, my views of that have changed dramatically. Of course I can still offer the same level of support to my patients; sometimes more! When you work in an acute setting, you may be more active and involved with a patient, but often for a shorter time and in a situation that is not normal. Now I realise that in our clinic setting I'm able to get a more holistic view of a person, as I'm there with them as they travel through the different milestones of life. I guess at an out-patient clinic we see more of a patient's daily life rather than a small and volatile fragment.

•   When I was considering a career in palliative care I remember a psychiatrist teaching me a wise strategy for patient interactions that I still utilise today. She suggested coaxing your patient to get the issue that was giving them the most grief off their mind first, as this would then allow a clearer mind to discuss the ensuing issues. Leaving the hardest and scariest things until the end of the consultation, where you wouldn't be left with a lot of time to solve other problems, wasn't going to help anyone. Basically, just go straight toward the elephant in the room first!

•   And finally, learn from other nurses and find support. For me, having the support from my international colleagues has been life-altering. I literally could not stop crying throughout my speech when I was awarded the inaugural International MS Nursing Leadership award; I felt seen. I would like to thank each and every one of them, but especially June Halper, whose unequivocal support to me and my regional colleagues has shaped the specialty of MS nursing in my region. And thus, I am committed to paying it forward.

ASTRID SLETTENAAR

Borne, eastern Netherlands

My job makes me exceptionally happy.
In fact, I think it's (almost) perfect....

....

I think in a way, MS nursing chose me. I had to take a break from the physical work of ward duties about eighteen years ago when I was 34 weeks pregnant with my second child. A colleague of mine had been asked by a neurologist to assist in establishing a MS out-patient clinic in Enschede and she asked if I would join her; from that point on I haven't turned back! Since that very first day at the clinic, I couldn't imagine being more enthusiastic about my career and I love that I meet inspirational patients and pioneering practitioners week in, week out.

I grew up in the Netherlands, in the east of Holland near the German border. After high school I commenced a Bachelor of Nursing and upon graduating, immediately started in the neurology ward at Medisch Spectrum Twente, one of the largest non-academic hospitals in the Netherlands. Then in 2003, a little more than five years after I began in general neurology, I started specialising as a MS nurse once a week. I don't think I ever imagined that working this single day a week in MS would lead to nearly two decades being passionately immersed in the field.

Then after a year of working with the team at the MS out-patient clinic, I decided to pursue a Master of Nursing, which two years later awarded me the nurse practitioner's certification and allowed me to work in multiple sclerosis research teams, perform physicals and also prescribe medications. In fact, the expanded responsibilities that obtaining my Master's afforded me was great; there was just so much more I could do for people with MS.

I clearly remember the very first day I worked in the MS clinic. Just seeing how enthusiastic but also independent those nurses were and the dedication they would show in striving for the perfect care of their MS patients was amazing. I could really see the difference between what they were doing within a clinic setting – in contrast to a hospital environment – and it was something I knew I wanted to embrace from the beginning.

The clinic was where I first learned to work independently and run cases and projects by myself. The team I work in every day is quite comprehensive and filled with a variety of people with varying expertise, so it's quite an inspirational environment to work in: We all know our areas of strength.

When I transitioned into an outpatient clinic, there was certainly plenty of other adjustments to make in my nursing style too. In my early days on the neurology ward, I was used to focussing very much on the patients, obviously for many, many days. But going into a clinic, you have to learn to use your time in a different way. You may only see patients for an hour at a time, but our natural tendency as nurses is to want to fix anything we can – which is a lovely trait to have! But within the environment of the clinic, I had to learn to do it in a different way. I had to learn to prioritise and really hone in on the particular issue my patient was bringing to that appointment.

And while – as out-patient nurses – we might spend less time each day with patients, we'll instead spend more cumulative time with a patient over the years and it gives us the opportunity to really get to know people and hear their stories. I absolutely love that part of my job and I think this sort of interaction with my patients suits me better than the style I needed to cultivate as a ward nurse.

At the Medisch Spectrum Twente, I have around 350 MS patients under my care throughout the year. Many of these people live close by. With a population of approximately 17 million, the Netherlands may be considered a small country, but we have more than a hundred major hospitals, so people don't have to go too far at all to find good medical attention. At my hospital, we have eleven neurologists, two of who specialise in MS. We also have a rehabilitation centre close by and they have built a comprehensive MS team of physical and occupational therapists and a specialist rehabilitation doctor and psychologist. So I believe that the care for people with MS in my region – the Eastern Netherlands – is very well-resourced.

***

Time brings clarity.

Understandably, getting told you have MS is a life-changing event. And those early years are such an uncertain time for the newly diagnosed and their family because the diagnosis itself is one thing but determining how active the disease is takes time and monitoring.

When they are diagnosed, the patient will invariably have many, many things on their mind, but time does bring clarity and I nearly always see a big difference in people twelve months later. They have different thoughts, they are starting to think about healing and even thriving. And that's not to say that some people don't need a lot of coaching along the way, but I do see that time brings clarity. So I consider one of my most significant roles in their journey is getting them through those crucial first twelve months and then we can tackle the residual issues as they need.

One thing I've come to truly believe is that creative people struggle less. It's something I witness every day. I think if something is taken from you, and you set about to find a way to compensate or alternate, then you're able to just move on. The patients I've met who exhibit creativity don't tend to see problems; they simply don't want to live life thinking about a set of problems. They want to create a solution and move on. And I recognise this coping mechanism displayed in an array of situations, from trying to find a better way to open a soda can right through to sexual dysfunction. I see and hear about some very imaginative solutions!

And while creativity is one thing, the temperament of perfectionism is another entirely! I've read a few times that a lot of people diagnosed with MS would have characterised themselves as being a 'type A' personality. And I find that the patients I might characterise as perfectionists can often struggle initially with the diagnosis of MS. As neurologists and nurses, we can't actually explain what causes MS, how or even if the disease will progress and what symptoms may or may not manifest. And I think that lack of certainty or control can frustrate the MS perfectionists.

Creative people have an easier time accepting the 'big picture' scenario and don't expect all the answers to be in front of them. They struggle with far fewer conflicts. I think ideally, you want to find a balance between the two characteristics. In fact, at our clinic, we use the word 'balance' all the time and in so many contexts. Obviously, we use the word to denote the physical context in describing a symptom, but we also would like to see our patients find a mental, psychological, emotional and lifestyle balance. The notion of balance means different things to different people and in this sense, we can only guide; it would be difficult to give a concrete 'how to' guide to each patient on how to find their own balance. Contrast this with the fact that we can give much more concrete direction when prescribing a disease modifying therapy (DMT) for a patient, because we have a greater medical understanding of matching people to treatments. It must be hard for people living with MS to reconcile when to trust what their medical team is recommending or prescribing and when they need to figure out the solutions themselves. And from our point of view, there is certainly no 'one size fits all' approach either.

But it's that very quandary that makes my job so interesting, and every day brings a different patient with a different journey to go on.

I'm a very creative person myself and since an early age, I had a tendency – or maybe a determination – to adapt things around me to solve problems. My sister tells a story how, as the youngest kid in our group of local friends, I was too small to ride a bike. Did it stop me from hanging out with my friends? No! I looked at the challenge from another perspective and instead learned how to run very fast so as I could keep up with everyone as they rode their bikes.

And still I'm always thinking about how I could help a person dealing with MS live better and in a creative way. I quickly identified that cooking is one of the first things that people with MS often give up when they're fatigued. I think this is so sad, because cooking can be therapeutic, but it can also be a great way to bring the family together. I also think giving the gift of your own cooking to those people around you who provide support can make a beautiful and heartfelt gift. It's very personal. So I worked on creating a cook book that guides people in how to adapt their kitchen, adapt recipes for easier preparation and also how to better manage their symptoms in the kitchen, such as fatigue, numbness, sensory or cognitive disturbances, dizziness and even dysphagia. The cookbook has been distributed all over the world and translated into Dutch, English, German and Czech.

I think by creating resources like this, we are finding a positive way to talk and also live with a chronic illness.

For me, the most inspiring MS patients are those that just work around their challenges; they find a way to cope with anything that is thrown at them. I know that for many of these people, every day would be full of comprises and having to remain flexible, but they just seem to get on with things rather than dwell on what they can't do.

The most common questions patients ask me are the questions fuelled by fear. They want to get an idea of how the disease will progress in their bodies and what life will look like five and ten years down the track. And of course, the onset of a new symptom nearly always raises fear and many questions. And new symptom onset can be frustrating for both the patient and the health team because often there's not too much we can do. The patient will feel the need to do something about it immediately – or at least consult with us immediately – to allay their fear. Treating these things that we are so uncertain about is the most difficult thing about treating MS because there is just so much that we can't answer yet.

And learning how to talk about that fear was one of my great challenges in the early years of my nursing career. I came to realise it could be more important to address that fear and uncertainty a patient was feeling than the symptom itself. This realisation changed the approach I took in my consultations.

***

Undertaking my Master's in nursing certainly accelerated my practical and professional education but also really helped me build greater life skills to help me in the clinical environment. Just as we try to guide our patients to find a sense of balance, so too did we learn the same skills to mitigate stress and burnout. We were taught that to find our own balance and indeed protect our own mental and emotional wellbeing that we needed to take off our figurative white coat the moment we left the hospital. I know many colleagues find it difficult to do but I don't personally have any problems with it and don't take my patient's challenges home with me.

In fact, I have a process where I like to let go of my day's stress as I'm on my way home. It's a process of reminding myself who owns the pain or the problem I'm experiencing. By recognising that I don't 'own' the problem, it's easier for me to leave that problem at the clinic where it belongs and where I can most efficiently deal with it.

I know that I can't do my job properly – for the greatest benefit of my patients – if I don't take time out for myself. I can also clearly distinguish the difference between being empathetic or unduly taking on someone else's problem. As a nurse, we are empathetic people, but taking on someone else's burden is not our job. We have to maintain a certain distance and also create a mental break from our patients so as we can keep our own sense of perspective and give advice that is unbiased. We have greater ways we can help than taking on a problem that is not ours to take on. I often see the partners or parents of people with MS who fall into this issue. They take on the burden of MS rather than being 'part' of the support and they lose perspective and objectivity in solving the challenges at hand because of it.

My Master's degree also taught me to better communicate with the neurologists I work with. This advanced education gave me the skills and vocabulary to be able to speak their language and this has assisted greatly in how I can do my work.

The nurse practitioners I know are pioneers and innovators, yet some of the neurologists we work with tend to take a more traditional approach to treatments, which can understandably create some clashes. It can be frustrating when we present ideas for a patient's care to a neurologist and get told that we are going 'too fast' or that they need more time to consider things. Our passion and motivation can sometimes take a hit when our progressive nature doesn't match that of the neurologist.

One example of this is that I have a vision for turning our outpatient clinic into a comprehensive centre for MS care. We have an excellent rehabilitation centre nearby and I see the tremendous work undertaken by the comprehensive centres in the east of Holland. I know the quality of care we provide at our out-patient clinic is exceptionally high but when I presented my ideas to expand and consolidate our service offering to the neurologists, they were very cautious and reticent. Maybe one day.....

The introduction of new DMTs onto the market is also something I think scares them, whereas I want to know as much as possible about new treatments in hope we might find a better match for some patients and can also be supportive in offering the full range of treatments available.

The very first neurologist I worked with had an enormous impact on my career and also taught me a lot about life in general. I was quite young when I transitioned from the neurology ward to the MS outpatient clinic and there were certainly times I was nervous about my role in the new environment. I worried if I was experienced enough for the responsibilities I had to undertake, but this neurologist would have a little bit of wisdom – a life quote – for everything! He was very supportive mentoring me through my Master's and also taught me to focus on the areas I could control rather than the things I couldn't. He was instrumental in getting me on the right track to where I am now.

And fostering great communication amongst our neurologists has been very important for me. We have eleven neurologists in our hospital and whilst I have the most interaction with our two neurologists who specialise in MS, working well with everyone is important – particularly as a nurse practitioner – so as I can create the best care and treatment plan for my patient.

One of the greatest joys of my job is being able to get to know my patients through the conversations we have. I feel that getting to know them better can only help the care I provide. But over the past few years, our consultation times have been shortened as we endeavour to maximise the nursing resources. We used to allocate one hour for each consultation, but this has now been reduced to 35 minutes.

The shorter consultations were hard to adapt to at first but one thing it has done is provide a sense of focus to the sessions. In fact, my patients are sort of trained now to come into my sessions with a list of things they want to discuss so we can make the most of our time. From my point of view, I've also had to rationalise what I can achieve within the allocated time, and this may mean referring a patient onto a specialist far quicker than I would have in the past. An example of this might be referring a patient with mental health requirements to a psychologist.

In one way that is a good thing, because it forces me to focus primarily on the medical care I can provide, but on the other hand, I am still a MS nurse and I can't help but want to provide holistic care and talk through things with a patient myself.

I think a lot about creativity and perspective and trust and fear. I believe that trust is the opposite of fear and that trust and hope are the most important things in dealing with a chronic illness like multiple sclerosis. The advice I often give to my patients is that we may not know with certainty what is going to happen whilst living with MS; but no matter what your body will do or how it might change, you must have trust that you will be okay. You will learn to handle this, and you will find solutions. You are not alone.

My hopes for the future treatment and management of MS:

• My hope for the future of MS is to find out what causes the disease. If we can understand how it begins, I think we have a chance to find out how to unravel it.

• We know that people who get onto a DMT earlier do better in managing their MS. Diagnosing MS has also become much better as the capability and precision of our MRI technology has advanced. And while we might not know what causes MS or have a cure yet, we still know so much more about the disease than ever.

• I hope that in the near future we can fully customise the DMT to our patients and predict the course of the disease and plan for and provide specific symptom management.

My advice for nurses beginning their career:

• Listen, listen, listen!

• It may be hard for action-oriented nurses but listening carefully and intently will ensure you don't immediately jump to actions and interventions that may not necessarily be exactly what your patient needs at that particular point in time.

• We have such a great network of MS nurses and nurse practitioners in the Netherlands and I always feel re-assured that I can reach out to them whenever I have a perplexing problem. It's great for other nurses to ensure they have a similar support network.

• As a board member of the MSNICB I'm presented with the opportunity to speak at a lot of conferences and I find the inter-national network of nurses very inspirational and tremendously important for my own professional development. Hearing how my colleagues do things in other countries is very fascinating.

JENNIFER BOYD
Toronto, Canada

A pioneer in the field of paediatric MS nursing.

According to the International Paediatric MS Study Group (IPMSSG), paediatric MS is defined as two or more episodes of central nervous system (CNS) demyelination in a patient younger than age 18, separated by more than thirty days and involving more than one area of the CNS. The National Multiple Sclerosis Society (NMSS) have estimated 8,000 to 10,000 children in the Unites States have MS, while another 10,000 to 15,000 have experienced at least one symptom suggestive of MS.

To put that into a global perspective, studies suggest that approximately 5% of all MS cases affect the paediatric population, primarily teens between the ages of 13 and 16, whilst MS in children under age 10 occurs in less than 1% of all cases of MS. Up to ten percent of patients diagnosed with MS may have had their first symptom before 18 years of age.

***

I was born in Kitchener, Ontario but grew up in London, Ontario – all within a few hours of Toronto, where I would eventually reside. Around late high school I realised how interested I was in medicine and it was really just a matter of debating whether I could see myself becoming a physician or a nurse. But I was ultimately drawn to nursing and I successfully applied to a nursing programme at the University of Western Ontario and it's been opening wonderful doors for me ever since.

I started my career in general paediatric nursing before working in public health nursing for a couple of years. Then an interesting role involving paediatric rehabilitation at the Easter Seals Society arose, allowing me to care for children with physical disabilities. My time at the Easter Seals evolved to encompass a variety of responsibilities, including home-care nursing, family education coordination and also some senior management duties.

Then in 1994, I decided to undertake my master's degree, focussing on paediatric neuroscience nursing with a qualitative research study on chronically ill children's perceptions of coping with repeated hospitalisations. During my master's, I took a clinical placement in neurosciences at The Hospital for Sick Children in Toronto, which fit perfectly with what I'd been doing for the previous four or five years.

Just as I was finishing up this placement, it turned out that a colleague I'd been working with was changing positions and urged me to apply for her job in the neurology clinic. Well, I got the job at SickKids and the rest is history!

The Hospital for Sick Children was inspired by the example of the Great Ormond Street Hospital in London, United Kingdom. During the spring of 1875, an eleven-room house was rented for $320 a year by a Toronto women's bible study group led by humanitarian Elizabeth McMaster. The group set up six iron cots and declared open a hospital 'for the admission and treatment of all sick children.'

Some 145 years and several moves and expansions later, SickKids – as it has come to be known – has over 350 beds and is internationally recognised as a major paediatric teaching hospital. In 2018, SickKids had over 16,200 inpatient admissions throughout the year, with a further 239,000 outpatient clinical consults.

For me, there was never any question that I wanted to work in the field of paediatrics, and I took every opportunity available throughout my early training to build on my experience; even vacation jobs would see me working summer camps! Working with children was just where my heart lay.

***

I'd only been working as a clinical nurse specialist for a few years when – in the late 1990s – our team found ourselves in a situation at the neurology clinic at SickKids where we had a number of children being diagnosed with MS. We were seeing that the paediatric neurologists would refer their patient onto the adult neurologists who specialised in MS. The adult MS neurologists would then confirm the diagnosis and suggest treatment but they then weren't feeling comfortable having paediatric patients in their care because treating and managing a disease or chronic situation in just about anything is different for a paediatric patient compared to an adult one. At the time, disease modifying therapies (DMTs) for MS were relatively new and one of the largest concerns was how to adapt treatments tested and developed for adults across to a child. There's certainly a grey area to all of this when we talk about a cohort of MS patients who are late teenagers, but the divide was rather large otherwise.

Families of these paediatric MS patients were instead turning to the Canadian MS Society for further information and support and the Society eventually approached one of our paediatric neurologists to see if we could develop specialised services for the kids. Serendipitously, we had a new paediatric neurologist joining us and it seemed like a great fit to have her create a paediatric MS clinic. So from that point on, myself and another clinic nurse formed a small team which was the foundation of the first paediatric MS clinic in the world. It was an exciting time knowing we could better support these families and provide a high level of expertise in a very unique situation.

Our clinic today now encompasses two paediatric neurologists (who specialise in neuro-inflammatory cases), a nurse practitioner, a clinic nurse who coordinates a great deal for us and also consulting specialists in psychiatry, psychology, social work and also a paediatric rehabilitation centre that can support our families.

Other locations, particularly in the US, became very interested in what we were doing and soon we had a few other places around the world who could also provide support in paediatric MS. There's now a paediatric MS interest group alongside a more formalised consortium of centres who can assist with care and in providing a greater range of treatment and disease management options.

***

In the here and now...

People often shake their head in shock that MS can affect kids so young and will wonder about the diagnostic and treatment process. At SickKids, how a paediatric patient comes to find us is probably very similar to the adventure that adults take in becoming diagnosed with MS and eventually meeting their own clinical care team. Some children are referred directly to the clinic with either a suspected or confirmed diagnosis of MS and others come under my care because they've been admitted to the hospital's emergency care with a severe flare and will then go on to be diagnosed with MS.

If I'm meeting a patient and their family for the first time in a hospital ward environment, then I'm likely to only introduce myself initially and explain what it is I do. I just don't feel that anyone can absorb too much information in those early days, so it's probably more important for me to simply show some support and help the family come to terms with the hospitalisation and recovery process after that first flare. There's just too much shock to deal with... the shock of how the flare manifested, the shock that it's serious enough for hospitalisation and then the shock that your child potentially has multiple sclerosis. At least if I've introduced myself from the onset, the family feel like they know a familiar face at the clinic, and that familiarity potentially makes it easier when we need to start some more serious dialogue around MS and begin introducing educational resources.

But more often than not, the first time I'm meeting the kids is as newly diagnosed patients within the clinic setting. I'm usually my team's 'go to' person to spend a lot of time with the families in those early days so as we can talk about different treatment options and disease management resources and just generally help people in getting their mind around the many facets of MS.

As I mentioned before, the pathway to diagnosis for a paediatric patient is much the same as that for an adult patient. That initial flare may have landed them in hospital under emergency care or similarly a variety of concerns – say optic neuritis or loss of sensation – may have led to MRI's and further investigation by a neurologist. Either way, it can be tricky to sift through some of the symptomatic indicators at times. Children don't always know how to identify, let alone explain, how they're feeling something that would be considered abnormal. And having them recall how long the symptoms have been troubling them, or the onset of any abnormalities, can also be a little fuzzy.

The work-up we undertake to rule out other possibilities is quite rigorous in paediatric patients for this very reason. I liken it to putting together many pieces of a puzzle, and that's generally the analogy I'll use to describe the process to a family. Often, we're moving several of the puzzle pieces around, flipping some pieces over and then along comes that critical piece of the puzzle that allows us to see the big picture with clarity.

The wait for a confirmed diagnosis is because we're being as certain as we can in ruling out other possibilities; there's just so many diseases that you would only see in children but not in adults. And whilst we are getting better and faster at diagnosing MS in adults, the world of paediatric MS is still largely trying to catch up to adult diagnostics because there's just far less case studies or research to guide us in the anomalies which are distinct in a paediatric diagnosis.

Do parents understand the scope of my role as the MS specialist nurse? I think that my role in talking about treatments and medications is an entry point for a lot of people to understand the part I play, and those conversations around treatments are then able to segue into a variety of different topics.

I'm careful to explain in my first meeting how we have an entire team working together to provide an overall health plan, including monitoring treatments and guiding them through the education of MS; and I particularly make mention that treatment management is just one part of what we do.

I also like to counsel the parents of my patients to give a name to what is being diagnosed. It's important that the children understand what they have is called 'MS' or 'multiple sclerosis' and not to be confused with something else they have heard, such as brain tumours or conditions that they may mistakenly associate with dying. This is especially relevant if children see how their parents are reacting to everything and leap straight to the conclusion that they might be dying. Portraying details to the children with clarity is quite important at this point. Obviously it can really depend on the age group we're dealing with, but I personally believe that being simple and open with the diagnosis from the onset can make things easier as we travel on this journey.

Disclosure of the diagnosis is an interesting topic for the MS patient, no matter the age, but there's certainly a lot of factors to consider in paediatrics. Who 'owns' the diagnosis and whose responsibility is it? Some children are mature enough to understand the consequences of people knowing that they are living with MS, some parents need to share the news to garner wider support and then there's so many combinations and considerations in between. We did a study that indicated the significance of sharing the diagnosis with close family and also those people who are important in the life of the parent and the child. A good example of this is the child's teacher. The teacher may be able to implement a range of very simple things that will make their pupil's experience in the classroom much more comfortable and accommodating of any symptoms. Or does a child's sporting coach need to be fed into the loop as well so as they can be conscious of managing symptoms of physical or heat fatigue when participating in sports? And parents may not even need to – or choose to – tell teachers and the like that their child specifically has MS but may instead just provide an understanding that they're dealing with health issues and particular symptoms need to be accommodated. It truly is a very personal issue for every patient and their family to address but I'm there to guide within the individual comfort levels and provide what I think are helpful examples.

I liken a kid's pursuit of schooling to that of an adult building a career or going to work. It's the kid's 'job' to go to school and get an education and so the issues of disclosure that kids with MS will face are actually very similar to those that adults might face in the workplace. And a kid's social life and peer group relationships also fit into the same scenario. These are all major spheres for a kid's development, and we want them to participate in all the things in life that satisfy and enrich – again much like an adult would – and we work hard to pave the way. So whether we give a name to the disease or not, or no matter how invisible the disease may be, we want everyone who's involved in the child's life to know how to respond to some of the challenges that MS brings.

I think the diagnosis is hardest for the parents at the beginning of the journey. It's very likely that a parent's pre-existing vision of MS is a person who is somewhat progressed and disabled, possibly in a wheelchair. And we endeavour to change that vision and explain that many, many people live active and full lives without any severe disability. Essentially, we want to help parents understand that the role of the medical team is to help their child live as normal a life as possible.

And the parents are always thinking more towards the future, whereas a younger child and the teenagers are definitely in the here and now. The kids simply want to make sure they can hang out with their friends and most of them don't want to miss any school either. I actually hear a lot of kids bemoaning the fact they have to go to a medical appointment because they don't want to miss school!

I think in many ways, kids are more resilient than adults. I see how when a life-changing diagnosis such as MS is thrust onto a kid, that often their biggest concern is just wanting to get on with life and trying to be as normal as possible. They have different priorities in those much younger years I guess, and I see them striving pretty diligently to just do what it is they want to do, be that go to school, play sports or simply keep friendships 'normal.' And because of this, kids might be quicker than adults to adopt work-arounds in symptom management. I had one patient who was intent on playing softball as much as she could because it was something she loved. When summer came, it was a no-brainer for her to don a cooling vest so she could get out onto the field and play and not let the heat knock her around so much.

And sharing stories about how other kids their age adapt and get on with things is absolutely an important part of my toolkit in caring for paediatric patients. The sort of advice I'll give is to recognise who their support network is and who can help them along this journey. I also love to reinforce that they can – and in fact it's important to – live as normal a life as possible. And we have a whole team of people who can help them with that pursuit!

Our centre worked with the MS Society of Canada to create a MS Summer Camp where kids living with MS could all get together and do normal camp activities, but they had the camaraderie of other kids in a similar situation. They could share stories and experiences and find comfort that someone else knew what they were going through. Often these kids with MS find that they're the only one in their community living with the condition, so for them to meet others from across North America also living with MS brings a touch of normalisation. The kids just love the camp and I daresay it could be life-changing for them to feel this support of peers.

***

There's clearly so many different factors to take on board when treating paediatric MS patients. You find yourself being forever vigilant at how the medical, emotional and psychological traits all intertwine whilst also knowing that our breadth of knowledge in any of these lacks the research and resources for the same traits experienced in adult MS.

And that's not a criticism of any particular system but simply an observation; and for me, it's meant building up a lot of skills and experience to fill the resource gaps between paediatric and adult MS. Certainly, a long career in paediatric nursing has contributed to those skills in a major way, as I've had many years of supporting parents and children through a range of difficult diagnoses. And in paediatric neurology in general there's just so many difficult situations. So I came into MS with a bit of a built-in skill set, but what I find now is it's the kids and parents dealing with MS who are teaching me what they need to know. Outside of our clinic sessions, I'll regularly get phone calls about other issues and that's generally where I'll start picking up on the themes that keep repeating and the type of information that families really seem to want and need. Isn't it funny how the heart of the issue is often realised in a less formal way?

In the early days after setting up the MS clinic, I was usually urged to meet with families very quickly after the diagnosis to discuss treatments. But over time, I came to realise it wasn't the best approach. After twenty years of doing this, I know inherently that my first contact needs to be a simple introduction and show of support, which then allows time for the diagnosis to be absorbed. At that introductory meeting we'll organise a follow up session to discuss a range of things – including possible treatment options – but I fundamentally believe that allowing time and space after the news of diagnosis is advantageous.

Completing my master's research presented me with great opportunities to pick up on a lot of themes and information that would ultimately shape how I performed my consultations. Areas such as disclosure are a good example of this. I guess undertaking the research gave me the time to talk with families and patients in a deeper way and understand what they needed. While on the job learning is so very valuable, obviously when you're undertaking research, the research is both the focus and reason for the discussion and for me, it gave me that opportunity to really zero in on certain topics.

My research also taught me about how people cope. Bringing all of the learnings from my research into the spotlight gave me a great body of information that I could use to explain how different people deal with different situations. And in many ways, what I was telling my patients and their families was no longer anecdotal but instead now had a base of evidence to it.

And at the end of the day, people don't want to feel alone. They will find re-assurance knowing others have gone through the same or similar experience. And my research was able to show them that. And the other skill my research gave me was a more finely tuned sense of what people were thinking, even if they weren't saying it verbally. This skill alone was helpful in judging where a family's headspace was and how I could sequence the information or resources that needed to be covered for maximum effect and benefit.

***

Kids are pretty smart...

Educating our paediatric patients on MS symptoms is a different challenge to how adults comprehend the symptoms and then go on to develop symptom management techniques. But kids are pretty smart. Often smarter than we give them credit for. We may use different words for things, but they still get it.

Take a symptom such as anxiety. We may probe to ask the kids if they're feeling worried or sad, and how often that might be, and if it might change how they do things during the course of their day? Or cognitive symptoms; we might talk to our patients about how they feel trying to memorise things at school or concentrating on things throughout the day and again, how these challenges arise and how it might change their experience at school. Basically, we aim to relate the various symptoms to what they're living with at the time. And this can be tricky, because the kids are still developing in themselves, even without the experience of MS. When adults are diagnosed, they're generally pretty developed, hence why we often say that MS hits you in your prime. But kids are a whole different ball game. I've found that if we do a bit of goal-setting with the paediatric patients from the beginning, this can help us build a vision for what a 'normal' life looks like for them and set some goals around that, because aiming for a regular life is what we are trying to achieve in providing symptom management and MS treatments.

I think my role as a MS nurse generally encompasses more elements of counselling or guiding paediatric patients on how to live well with MS rather than dealing with many physical aspects of disability. And the other area not to be overlooked is the psycho-social elements of paediatric MS because it truly is a family thing. I could absolutely find myself providing significant support to the parents in those early days of diagnosis as they're the ones feeling the strain of dealing with the burden of disability and we need to channel the support and resources there initially. It's often in the early days that parents struggle with feelings of guilt and even query whether it's something they did to cause the MS. They may be beating themselves up that they didn't pick up on the symptoms of MS sooner and they'll feel further guilt over that too. Then there's also the burden of supervising treatments and how the parents can adequately provide support, right through to feeling as if the vision they had for their child's future has been crushed.

All these worries accumulate and if we can help the families through this first, we can then pave a way for a clearer treatment and management plan.

And then somewhere different in the mix, we have teenagers who won't necessarily want to talk about any of this. They're certainly comprehending of the gravity of the situation and either don't want to cause concern for their parents or just aren't ready themselves to confront dealing with a disease that is life changing.

Let's be honest: Being a teenager with MS is a particularly challenging situation. Relapses and MS symptoms such as physical and cognitive fatigue may cause teens to miss school and cut back on social activities, or simply feel 'different' from their peers at a time when they are just trying to fit in.

Anecdotally I think that the younger the patient is, the more compliance there is to a treatment plan, perhaps because you have a parent who is essentially telling the child to take their meds or do a particular thing every day. Then other times we see kids who are extremely motivated to adhere to a treatment plan. It may be they have a different type of support around them or are driven to achieve something in particular.

I find the earlier we can have a patient understand the correlation between how their motivation to consistently take a treatment or do a therapy will affect their success of living with MS, the greater chance we have to achieve a treatment plan adherence. Essentially the kids just need to embrace as soon as possible that medications and therapies are part of living with MS.

Where I've seen the medication adherence issues become more problematic are among adolescent patients who rebel because they want to feel normal and may not understand or believe the medications are necessary.

Drs Mah and Thannhauser, researchers from the University of Alberta, noted in their paper titled 'Management of multiple sclerosis in adolescents – current treatment options and related adherence issues' that "Adolescents' sense of omnipotence, cognitive limitations in assessing risks, and relative inexperience with long-term consequences (especially with an 'invisible' disease like MS) may lead to the belief that they do not need to follow the treatment plan."

The researchers go on to explain "the social systems within which these young patients live also influence their ability to adhere to treatment regimes. Specifically, peer relationships are of critical importance during adolescence. Treatment regimens can have negative implications for peer relationships, such as interrupting or restricting social activities and changing lifestyle. Injection-site reactions and side effects of high dose corticosteroids can also alter physical appearance, resulting in adolescents becoming more self-conscious of their bodies. Feelings of being different can lead to social withdrawal. Pre-existing family dysfunction or other stressors may restrict much needed caregiver support and impede adolescents' follow-through with treatment regime."

As a paediatric MS nurse, I find I'm contacted about pretty much any symptom that's going on, whether it's logically related to MS or not. I think it emanates from a paediatrician or a GP wanting to refer to a specialist MS nurse because they don't know enough about MS – let alone MS in kids – and won't have a clear answer themselves. And I guess I'm glad for the opportunity to work alongside other health care professionals so as we can modify or advise on health matters to keep our patient just generally living as a healthy human, even whilst dealing with MS.

Striving to live as healthy humans is the same proposition in MS whether you're an adult or an adolescent. Whilst adult patients may be counselled on maintaining good heart care health, weight management or stress and anxiety reduction, for paediatric patients we're aiming to promote a similar awareness of maintaining a healthy lifestyle, it's just that we'll phrase the objectives differently and instead talk about exercise and basic dietary guidelines and beneficial behaviours that promote good overall health.

**

Working the room

A key aspect of managing paediatric MS is adjusting the approach during the transition into adolescence and teen years. As the young patient matures, there is a need to encourage more independent decision-making and responsibility. Better adherence to therapy is linked to whether the young adult chooses to take responsibility for his or her own self-care and teens whose MS was diagnosed earlier in childhood may require some re-education about their disease, since much of the earlier education was directed toward the parents.

And undoubtedly teens and young adults will face new situations, such as deciding whether or when to disclose the diagnosis of MS to their friends, intimate partners, teachers, and employers. In addition, there are many new medical issues related to puberty and adulthood, including birth control and family planning, and expanded exposure to substances such as cigarettes, drugs, or alcohol.

Yes, that transitionary period from childhood to adolescence can be tricky for so many reasons and living with MS can definitely make it even trickier!

I experience mixed feelings when someone I've been caring for transitions into adult care. Naturally I become quite attached to my patients and care about their future and I also recognise our team at the paediatric MS clinic provides a familiar environment for the patient and family. But I inherently know that part of the growing up process is for my patients to start being treated like young adults, particularly when it comes to health care. And you can't forget that as young adults, the patients also have greater access and choices in the medications and clinical trials that might be available to them in managing MS.

I'm always careful to present the transition from our paediatric care into adult care as a positive occasion, re-assuring the patients that there are great nurses and neurologists on the 'other side.' I might also coach them a little bit with the sorts of questions they could be asking their new health care team – basically just some small little tips to help them become used to the new faces and environment as seamlessly as possible.

And you have to keep in mind that when paediatric patients transition into adult care, they're typically very transient in nature anyway. You've only got to look at your own children or nieces and nephews and reflect how in their late teens you never really knew all that they were up to in school or sports or social activities, but you certainly recognised they were always on the move! These are kids who are trying to figure out their own lives as well and haven't settled into anything in particular yet.

In fact, I often find the transition is harder on the parents; their attachment to us is possibly a little stronger.

Because I've spent my entire career in paediatrics, I've learned that the intrinsic approach I need to have in treating patients is one of managing multiple relationships. There's the relationship I have with my patient and then the relationship with their parents. Basically,

I've learnt that I just need to 'work the room' and deploy a number of different communication styles to ensure the message is being heard and understood. Knowing your audience is critically important in treating paediatric patients and their families. It may sound like a big workload but it's all I've ever known and to me, it's just another part of the MS puzzle. The role of a paediatric nurse is fundamentally one that involves educating and guiding the whole family.

Perhaps the struggle comes later when – as the paediatric patients grow up – we have to adjust our approach a little because the patient requires a more sophisticated level of information and education than what we've provided in earlier years. There's a turning point where the younger patients start to realise that MS carries a lot of adult responsibilities and concepts. Some of the things we talk about when they're kids just don't mean that much at the time, but later in life – and with some education and maturity under their belt – all of a sudden some of this information starts to become a reality, such as 'labelling' the degree of MS. The concept of relapsing remitting MS may mean nothing to a twelve-year-old, it's just what they have; but as an eighteen-year-old, the label takes on a new life. And working out when the timing is right to start presenting a more sophisticated style of education and discussion can be delicate.

The types of knowledge and skills we help our adolescent patients develop might cover anything from being able to explain to health professionals the type of MS they have, along with greater awareness around symptom management and new symptom onset, signs of a relapse and also trying to guide patients when to recognise if something is MS-related or whether it's something else altogether. As those young adults become more independent, the necessity to start being self-aware becomes important, as they may no longer have their parents around as much to be vigilant or make determinations. I guess we're providing new communication skills for the patients as much as disease management skills. Even simple things such as how appointments get made or when to call a specialist on the telephone need to be discussed, as this has traditionally been under the purview of the parent and suddenly the young adults need to realise that this stuff doesn't just magically happen!

And it can't go unsaid that providing our paediatric patients a sophisticated level of awareness also means coaching the parents to allow and even embrace their child managing their own disease and that they need to let go a little to foster the transition.

***

You just have to really embrace that hopeful mindset in my line of work; to simply keep the bigger picture in mind...

I think just as patients need to work out what they can control and what they can't in MS, so too, do MS nurses experience the same challenge. I could get melancholy if I pondered how MS 'could' lead to a disease burden in my patients as they grow older, but I instead focus on what I can do now and what I can control now and that very hopeful difference I can make now.

And if feelings of sadness or hopelessness ever did enter my consciousness, I'm lucky that I work with an amazing group of people and I'm able to bounce ideas off them. We're all going through similar situations and being able to debrief with each other in those rough times is tremendously helpful. And finding some type of balance in life, which includes developing techniques to separate work and home life, is also incredibly important. I just don't think you can survive in our roles without this.

In the beginning there were certainly times of loneliness doing the work I do, because there just wasn't anyone else out there in paediatric MS nursing for a while! I had the support of many other specialist MS nurses with adult patients – and they absolutely got me through those patches of loneliness with their advice and resources and friendship – but sometimes I wasn't always sure of what I should be doing, especially when it came to treatment regimens; it could be exceptionally perplexing to navigate those areas. In paediatrics we work out our treatment dosages based on milligrams of medication per kilogram of patient weight, but multiple sclerosis treatments just don't work that way – they're designed to be one dose for all! And the neurologists and I had no experience in knowing how (or even if) to make dosage adaptations because our patient cohort was just too small for many experiences to have been captured.

But I was never scared as such, just more perplexed and concerned. I think paediatric medicine instils a very different set of skills in you from the beginning. When I was doing general paeds nursing we'd often have to manage and adapt medications that had been originally designed for adults to a child's individual situation. And in many situations, my colleagues and I were always trying to figure out the balance of what to treat and what not to treat in kids to ensure the optimal outcome. But MS can be a different beast...

I knew how to be a great paediatric nurse, so the challenge became melding paediatrics with what my adult MS nursing colleagues knew and adapting that to suit the unique circumstances of the kids I was caring for.

It might seem easy to lose hope or perspective at times, because what we're dealing with can be incredibly complex and fraught with emotion, but I tend to keep at the forefront of my mind that we are there to make a difference. We may not be able to change the diagnosis; we may not be able to cure the disease; but hopefully we can help our patient and their family find some positivity or comfort or resources to get on with life. I think you just have to really embrace that hopeful mindset in my line of work; to simply keep the bigger picture in mind rather than become embroiled in the minutia.

After thirty-five years of doing this, I reflect that being a pioneer in the field of paediatric MS nursing has given me the opportunity to connect with people from around the world and to travel to numerous cities and countries to share my knowledge. There is also immense professional satisfaction from creating a specialised clinic from the ground up, developing unique expertise, and making a difference for my patients and their families as they adapt to having a condition that has so many uncertainties.

And most simply, I feel inspired by the work I do. I get inspired to move ahead and make a difference for the patients I work with. And then when you see a resilience shining through and that the kids are getting on with life, it's nothing short of brilliant.

My hopes for the future treatment and management of MS:

•   Things have certainly evolved since I started working in MS twenty years ago but the fact that we even have treatments – let alone a few options – available for paediatric patients these days is amazing, given none at all existed until quite recently.

•   My hope is we can start seeing more precision medicine in MS and really start developing personalised treatment options that target a patient's specific situation.

•   I am very optimistic about the future of treatments given that we have so many more treatment delivery options now; we have a variety of injectables, orals and infusions, which provide better choices for patients.

•   In paediatrics we've learned so much more about the impact of MS on cognition and learning and fatigue, and this will help us tremendously in crafting tactics and management plans to help our kids have fulfilling school lives.

•   I'm buoyed by the positive impact of exercise for people living with MS. Kid's naturally love moving and being active, so if we can introduce this as a symptom management strategy early and we have evidence to back up the effects, then this could go a long way again in helping kids lead normal, healthy, active and involved lives. It's also very empowering for people living with MS to take control of their MS as soon as possible themselves.

My advice for nurses beginning their career:

•   Find your support network, both inside and out of work. A social life is really important!

• Develop (and maintain) interests outside of work that allow you to find a way to switch off and also just find a sense of balance. I love knitting (I'm a left-handed knitter!), Pilates and sinking my teeth into a great crime novel.

• Good time management techniques are important to learn so as you don't become solely focussed on work and disregard the necessity of having a life outside of work. Realising that generally those same worries or responsibilities are still going to be there the next day so taking some time out to refresh and recalibrate is an investment in yourself. It really is just a matter of knowing your priorities at any given point in time. I know earlier in my career I stayed far too long at work each day and it was an important lesson for me to realise that it was an unsustainable practice.

• Know the resources that are available to you, as there's always so much that can be learned.

• Take as many opportunities as you can to learn about MS and the field you're in. There are so many great ways to take on education now compared to when I started out twenty years ago. Webinars are much more accessible, and we have great online portals.

• Network with colleagues and other specialist nurses so as you can swap ideas and case studies.

• And don't forget to share your learnings and studies! We all cultivate our own areas of expertise and being able to pass on your pearls of wisdom is not only important but can be personally satisfying.

THERESE BURKE
Sydney, Australia

*"In Tibet we say that many illnesses can be cured
by the one medicine of love and compassion."
– the Dalai Lama.*

....

For the first time in my life, I'm going to have time out for me. I'll have time to think and recalibrate; working through my PhD is my focus at the moment and I'll be able to dedicate time to it and also just simply, dedicate time to me. It's a little bit scary to contemplate to be honest. After more than thirty years of being there for others – and passionately so – it's time to be there for myself.

But more about all of that later.....

***

I grew up in Dubbo, a small city in the Great Western Plains region of New South Wales, Australia. Whilst the website boasts of a diverse and exciting town with a population of some 40,000 people, sometimes it felt a lot smaller than that! I was the eldest child and have two younger sisters and a younger brother, Anthony. In fact, it was Anthony who probably drew me to the notion of nursing. He was born with achondroplasia, a form of dwarfism (or skeletal dysplasia), which affects bone growth. But growing up in a country town provided scant facilities for his care and I would help my mother and father with his treatments wherever I could. It really opened my eyes to the profession of caring for the first time.

I always had my heart set on going to university after high school but back in the early '80s it just seemed really expensive and was not an option. So instead, I set about finding a job where I got paid to learn something. To be honest, I was also keen to move to the city and away from the country, and nursing in Sydney seemed like the ideal option! Thirty years ago, nurses who were undertaking their training were given accommodation at the nurse's quarters within the hospital campus and it also paid me a small wage, so for someone fresh out of high school, it was a pretty good deal.

I don't remember ever having a burning yearning to be a nurse but the prospect of learning and finding a vocation away from country life ticked all the boxes for me. In fact, I don't think I ever really thought of where it would lead, beyond the fact that it was my ticket to doing something different.

I applied to two different hospitals in Sydney – North Shore and Westmead – logically choosing Westmead because their programme started sooner, thus getting me into my new life even earlier!

Westmead Hospital is a major tertiary hospital in Sydney. Opened in 1978, the 975-bed hospital serves a population of 1.85 million people and is a teaching hospital of Sydney Medical School at the University of Sydney, making it one of the largest health and hospital campuses in Australia.

Three years later, I finished my general training in Westmead and applied to go into the respiratory-based high dependency ward, which was the ward I particularly loved. Any other facility would have considered the unit an Intensive Care Unit (ICU), but

Westmead is such an enormous hospital that we had many speciality areas similar to this particular ward. I loved the intense nature of the environment and some of those nurses I started with in that ward remain life-long friends.

But it was a ward that was as scary as hell because people were dying on a daily basis; essentially, if you didn't need a ventilator to breathe but still needed intensive care, then you would have been put on this ward.

And so started my fascination with this field…

I ended up spending several years on the high-dependency ward, even extending my training to become a respiratory nursing consultant. I thought I had found my dream job, however about nine months into the new role, I fell pregnant with my first child. I inherently knew I wouldn't want to work full time after the birth of my daughter, so I began to look around for part time nursing work within Westmead. I was put in touch with the doctor who was in charge of the allergy service who needed a nurse to work part-time to manage an asthma trial for a new drug treatment. My experience on the respiratory ward made it a perfect fit. This temp role eventually led me into the world of immunology and little did I know then I would end up some thirty years later where I am today.

Everything seems so serendipitous but still, I can't imagine my career path turning out a different way. Looking back, I sometimes wonder if the attraction to forging a path in immunology came off the back of finding the world of respiratory medicine – and by default palliative care – so acute; I wonder if I was subconsciously wanting to move away from the dire nature of the ward before it had a greater impact on my disposition?

Over time, my role at Westmead evolved and eventually I settled into the position of coordinating the MS Clinic and the clinical trials unit. This role provided a perfect mix of clinical research work and patient-focussed consultations. Whilst the role had a research title, the sessions in the clinic ultimately ended up really taking over with the introduction of several new disease modifying therapies (DMTs) and the onerous patient care and supervision that these drugs and treatments needed.

Before taking on this research role, I'd had no experience or exposure to multiple sclerosis what-so-ever; I knew nothing at all about it. And again, I found this role in neuro-immunology by chance. The doctor I had previously been working with in the asthma trial left for another hospital, which was much further away and given my family commitment, I didn't want to commute the extended distance. However, she shared her office with a neuro-immunologist who was able to offer me a place on his clinical team.

And I have to admit – at that time – it was just a job. I was lucky because it was a job in the same department, I could retain the flexibility I had, which was important to me whilst I was raising a family, and I knew the ropes and a lot of the personalities I was working with. I literally thought 'what the hell. This will be just fine.'

When I started in my neuro-immunology research role, the job was to help build up a MS clinical trials unit. My previous experience working with allergy clinical trials lent itself to this pro-cess. The DMT's Lemtrada and Tecfidera were planning their trials in Australia for the first time and Westmead had a well-established infusion centre and great resources, so we knew it was the best place to trial these new treatments. I was more a clinical trial research nurse in those early days but even back then I could see we knew so little about how patients felt and what was going on at the coalface of their treatments. I felt there was just such a huge gap between the trials, the ensuing treatment delivery and the actual patient care; I couldn't help but think that what we were doing could be far more than a clinical trials unit. We could do some investigator-led research and nurse-led research and look at how to deliver a better patient experience and outcome and then use that information to change the way we treat and manage patient care.

But it was a different time back then. We didn't have email and the Internet, which made finding the right connections to establish the programme I had in my mind very difficult. And ironically, the people and expertise we needed may well have been out there because at this same time – and unbeknownst to me – Kaye Hooper had started the MS Nurses Australasia (MSNA) organisation and there would have been about fifteen or twenty members, but neither myself or the neuro-immunologist I was working with knew about the group. It wasn't until just a little while later when we did have better Internet access that I came across the International Organisation for MS Nurses (IOMSN) and discovered Kaye and the work she'd been doing in Australia. Can you believe this was all only about 15 years ago? We can't imagine a life without the web, but it was fairly inadequate back then, both in availability and the breadth of information, so we didn't rely on it like we do now.

The curse of discovering the MSNA and the IOMSN fellowships was that I became frustrated that we had amazing nurses all over Australia (and in fact the world) who were doing wonderful research and patient work, but nobody wrote about it or acknowledged it past the occasional conference lecture. The nursing and patient experiences weren't being shared and recorded to shape and inform other nurses, let alone the next generation.

Kaye asked me to take on the presidency of MSNA in 2010 so we could really build up the collation and sharing of clinical nursing research and patient treatment experiences. It became my consuming mission. At that time, I remember attending an annual MS nursing conference on the Gold Coast and realising that across the whole event, there were only three small poster presentations talking about clinical research and trials in MS; it was just so sad and frustrating to me that this vital area was not more recognised. Fast-forward to nearly a decade later and we have a lot greater acknowledgement and focus on the importance of the research within the clinic environment of MS. We're seeing a lot more articles being published internationally by nurse-led research and clinical teams and I can see that this broader dissemination of material is helping other nurses and clinics worldwide. There's just a greater emphasis now on sharing information or working out what information or research other teams need to be able to make a difference.

***

"Sometimes you can give, give, give and it's just not what your patient needs."

Somehow, I find myself fifteen years into my nursing career. I've traversed the specialties of high-dependency and respiratory to land in neuro-immunology and along the way married the man of my dreams, Troy – who I met on my very first day at Westmead – and also given birth to two amazing children, Lauren and Nicholas. Those years have held so many joyful moments but similarly, there's been plenty of challenging situations I've had to face and some days I would go home feeling utterly broken.

Despite initially being a little cavalier and even ambivalent about the role I found myself in, I fell in love with it almost immediately. It just felt like 'home' for me and I loved my work in a way that I'd never experienced before. I had the time to learn and largely taught myself everything I needed to learn. As I set about setting up the clinical trials unit, I was able to talk to patients for hours, as back then, we only had a few dozen regulars and I found myself with plenty of time available. That makes me laugh now, as we eventually ended up with over 600 patients, all requiring very different therapies and consultations and some days I barely had time to run to the loo!

Maybe because I've experienced both ends of the patient management spectrum – going from the luxury of very long and detailed conversations to then having to juggle a diverse patient roster that is bulging at the seams – I've been able to trial and then fine tune a variety of consultation techniques.

The most common, everyday situations I faced were the people who are accepting of their diagnosis, keen to get help, keen to be educated and just keen to know more. The type of questions they would ask when first diagnosed depended so much on their personality and the things in life that were inherently important to them. In the early days, the most commonly asked questions were how long until I'm in a wheelchair? How long until I lose function? How long have I got left? Back then, patients would almost see multiple sclerosis as a fast-moving illness and they would need a number or a timeframe.

These days it's different. Most people are just generally more aware about what MS is and what it isn't. These days, the questions are more around work, family and pregnancy. So, if my patient is a young female, then pregnancy or the ability to have a child and any possible hereditary aspects will always be of great concern.

The question of 'how do I tell my parents?' is always a big one and I preferred to tackle that query very early on. A partner or a friend might be there on the journey with them but often in that age group of 20, 30 and 40s, the person with MS is unsure how to tell their parents or friends about the diagnosis because it's so hard for them to get all the concepts together in their head, particularly when it's new; they're still getting over the fact that they've had an episode or a flare and all the chaos that situation brings, and then we're hitting them not just with the diagnosis and the possible treatment options for MS but then also the social impact.

So those very early conversations can cover everything from detailing the eleven-plus types of drugs, the potential side effects of those drugs – some of which may potentially kill you – to whether having a family is still an option through to how to tell family and friends, let alone the impact on a person's career and work options. It's easy to see why anyone would be over-whelmed.

And believe it or not, if I've got someone in front of me who is quite keen to learn all of this and take it on board, then that's a good day in the office.

The other end of the equation is people who are not dealing with the diagnosis or their flare very well at all. They're full of steroids from the methyl prednisolone treatment, which is colouring every-thing as well, and they're still looking backwards and contemplating 'what the hell happened?' In their mind they went out to watch a game of baseball and their vision went fun-ny and next thing they're in hospital being told they have an incurable disease.

And then in the middle, I'm dealing with people who had an episode and were then diagnosed and referred to me, but they've gone back to baseline and are no longer experiencing symptoms so in their mind they're okay. I would hear them say things like "I think it's gone now. I'm fine, so why are we still talking about this?"

But by far, the hardest situations for me to handle were with the patients who were not accepting or believing and full of anger. High anxiety levels were difficult too, but I became a lot better at handling those days by undertaking a lot of pre-appointment work to identify potential issues. I learned to start my consultations with the simple question of "Now... what do you know? Tell me what you think this is going to look like for you." I would really want to know how they're feeling first up rather than bombarding them with information and options. The other thing I learned to do differently, is that when people cried – which was often – I would ask them why they were crying. I remember one of the neurologists I was working with asking me why I would do that? Wasn't it obvious? But the answers would constantly surprise me, and it often set the scene for ensuing conversations. And that's where I discovered the fear of telling their parents was a big reason for people to get upset. They would always explain that they were okay with the diagnosis but feared the news would destroy their parents.

In the early days, I always had a consultation sequence that I really wanted to stick to, but then I realised my sequence was great for me, but not necessarily my patient. I worked out that if we first addressed all those issues that the patient considered paramount, then I could back-track to the clinical and practical information that I feel they needed to walk away with. It took a bit of trial and error to tweak my consultation sequence, but I now know that the patient and their family would be more accepting of the information because we'd discussed the huge thing that was weighing down their mind or clouding their perception; the things that would stop them from hearing anything I'd be saying anyway! And I think that's a sign of maturity in myself and my experience as an MS nurse to have adjusted my patterns like this.

The cases where there's a lot of anger are the ones I found the most difficult. On those days when I was feeling a bit broken, then I found it really tough to also deal with a patient's anger being thrown right back at me. It's so hard to help them when they're just not in a position to listen or take advice. On the one hand I totally understood where they were coming from and dearly wanted to help… but when it was thrown straight back at me, I didn't have the skills at that time to deal with the feelings this invoked.

There was once a patient that I'd gone over and above in dealing with their anger and frustration, and eventually a colleague pulled me up and explained that I needed to stop getting side tracked with this case as it wasn't fair that they were sapping so much time and energy. In fact, it had started to take away valuable time and energy from the work I was doing with our other patients. This patient simply was not listening to what I was saying and was also shopping around several clinics, holding out to get the response they wanted to hear. I eventually had to have a very hard discussion with this patient and explain that it wasn't good for her, but it similarly wasn't good for the other clinicians she was seeing. That whilst the answers to her treatment options may vary between different specialists, the MS was still MS and it simply wouldn't change. I desperately wanted her to understand that shopping around and perpetuating frustration and anger would simply add to her emotional load and it wasn't a healthy way to deal with the disease.

As my colleague sagely explained, "Sometimes you can give, give, give and it's just not what your patient needs."

***

The mind games of an unpredictable, chronic illness.

Working in multiple sclerosis has increased my awareness of what an invisible illness can be about and the mind games that an unpredictable, chronic illness can play in someone's life. It's probably forced me to forget my own woes from time to time and get on with helping others.

The hard part is when you've got to go searching for the tools to stock your psychologists' tool kit and if you're really beaten down it's hard to find what you need, because you don't actually know what you need! Over the last few years we've had a variety of experts come and speak to us at the MSNA about those various tools, such as setting boundaries, meeting challenges and guarding time and energy. And it's not hard to understand why those workshops are the most highly attended ones!

We've also set up groups through the MSNA where we can speak to each other about various challenges and also counsel one another via our individual experiences. But all in all, there is no training to deal with this. We depend on what we can teach ourselves.

There was a time when things got a bit much for me and I took myself off to see a psychologist, just to work through a few things. I realised I needed an outlet because I was going through a rough patch where I didn't enjoy getting up in the morning to go to work; and that's not me. And whilst the sessions with the psych were somewhat helpful, I've personally found greater value in the wisdom of the MS nurses around me.

You know what? The advice of my peers has always been stellar and often it revolves around someone reminding me that the situation is actually not about me and to first and foremost step back and take myself out of the situation.

I'm extremely grateful to have the support of those other MS nurses around me – who are all very strong people – and they have never let me down.

***

I don't really see a trend or expect a timeline in what questions a patient will ask when. The disease is so individual for everyone. As people continue to live with the disease longer, they start asking some of the harder questions – especially those that are concerned about how they're going to be when they're much older. With this cohort, I tend to guide them to under-stand that time can actually be their friend.

But early into the MS journey, I feel most patients just need time and space to process the diagnosis and then understand the symptom manifestation; allow things to settle a little bit. And then when things do return to some type of normal, I urge people not to sit around contemplating or waiting for symptoms to flare or exacerbations to happen, but rather that time is their best friend and they should use it to live life; to prepare and use that upswing to compen-sate for any downswings.

Even now, I would still allow the same amount of time in my consultations for someone who has been living with MS for one year, ten years, twenty years…no matter the stage the patient is at, there's just always other things. And you also need to incorporate the education of healthy aging into the equation as well. Regardless, I find there's always something else or we use the time to dig a bit deeper. But I can assure you that living with the disease longer doesn't minimise questions or conversation between the patient and myself.

And in that way, as MS nurses, we become a one stop shop: Our roles are also part psychologist, part councillor, part clinician, part medical interpreter, part social worker, part educator, part mediator…. and the list goes on.

And that enormous responsibility we're bestowed is truthfully one of my biggest personal frustrations. Our patients do come to us with a myriad of questions, conversations and needs but I simply can't solve all the problems. I CAN solve some of the problems but in the bigger scheme of things I can solve very little.

Another challenge that can cause frustration is when a patient doesn't tell the truth. I understand that each person may have their own reasons for fudging the truth – from embarrassment to cognition issues to the outright denial – but that lack of being forth-coming is such a hindrance to how we can assist. We're so often time-poor, but if I've been lied to or information has been with-held then I also feel like I've been put in a position of solving a problem that isn't solvable because I'm not getting the right information. There are days when I'm just so 'decision made' and 'problem-solved' out that the lack of truthfulness makes it really, really tough. It doesn't happen often, but when it does, it can be devastating.

And a lot of how we deal with patient responses and conversely, how a patient interacts with us, comes down to timing. It can be dependent on how they're feeling that day, whether we're dealing with them first in the morning when we're fresh, or whether they're the thirtieth patient we've seen for the day. It comes back to that old issue of how crucial time and timing is in managing this disease. There was a time in the early days of my career when we saw a record-breaking 18 patients in one day. Now on clinic day, 30 to 35 is the norm. We don't even really think about the patient load any longer; we just know we've got to dig deep.

At the MS clinic, I established a nurse-led clinic day so as we could have one day a week where we saw less patients but could give them more time. In particular, those patients who may have been at a critical juncture of their treatment or were newly diagnosed. It was the one day where I felt I could really problem solve in a more concentrated way. And this nurse-led day, and even the time we grab as a team here and there, are great for problem solving. But it's still always under pressure. It's never relaxed and systematic. It's reactive but still somehow (surprisingly) functional.

I know some other clinics prioritise that round table time to sit down as a team and problem solve the challenges presented. And I can't rate this highly enough as an effective management process. I guess no matter the format it takes, I've found that building and strengthening those bonds with your colleagues is crucial. We've all cultivated different strengths and I'll be the first to admit that there's times I can't see the forest for the trees, yet I'm surrounded with colleagues I trust, who can offer an alternative vision or solution. Similarly, there's times I know I lend a perspective to the more clinical or blunt members of our team. I think a great clinic is forged from a variety of points of view. And indeed, it can help us understand and solve very complex problems.

I genuinely feel that MS, more so than many other diseases, is such a group effort and the sooner that every member of that team – from the neurologist through to the clinic receptionist – realises the vital skills they can bring to the table to help our patients, (and help each other), the better off everyone will be. Every person in our clinic had a unique and individual role to play and they each contributed to a part of the patient's journey.

***

> *"In Tibet we say that many illnesses can be cured by the one medicine of love and compassion."*
> *– the Dalai Lama.*

Is there a burden in feeling like you can't have a bad day? Absolutely. The hand-wringing irony is that we give our patients the permission to have a bad day; to scream and shout and get the emotion out so as they can find a release and bounce back. But I just can't. On those days when I would go into the clinic and my head just wasn't really in the space, or when I was feeling a bit off because there's other things going on in life, I could never allow myself to show a bad day.

Maybe it's some of the psychology I learned a while back, but I learned to glue a smile on my face and just hope that it permeated through my body. Do I worry about dampening my personal emotions? Again, absolutely. And I've read how it can lead to mild depression. But the tremendous joy I get from being able to help people through the work I do simply takes over anything I might be feeling. And I think in more recent times as I became quite run down, I've given a lot of thought to how it's possible that I can love something so much yet sometimes don't feel very good about it?

At base level, I know I love what I do. And I will use that word every single time, because I do love it. But how do I deal with something that just isn't good for me at the moment? These feelings have probably been bubbling along for four or five years. I now know that I should have pulled back to part time work, which I didn't do because the patient load was so significant, but I should have prioritised myself a little while ago.

Another burden is that I constantly come up against problems that I don't know how to fix. And that also upsets me, and I struggle with it. But let's face it; there are a lot of problems that people will present with, that there just aren't any solutions for. And that's when I go to a beautiful saying from the Dalai Lama. "In Tibet we say that many illnesses can be cured by the one medicine of love and compassion."

And I think MS is a bit like that. Medicine is only part of the equation when you're dealing with the disease. So, what is left is compassion and kindness. I strongly believe if you treat the people in your care with compassion and kindness – even if you can't solve their problem – that is still the best thing you can do for them. I love his quote and it's a daily reminder for me in how to approach our work. You can't always fix heartache and you can't always solve disappointment. They're just things that people have to go through. I think because MS is such a multi-faceted disease, which can affect every part of your being, as nurses we tend to want to fix every part of the person. But it really isn't our job or our right to do that.

I truly feel that what we do is one of the most complex specialist nursing professions. More than anything else I can even think of. Before becoming an MS nurse, I was exposed to a myriad of other specialty areas and it's something I've discussed with other clinical nurse consultants and they all agree.

This is not a game of 'whose job is harder' but let me explain the comparison to you. A surgical nurse will likely be in a reasonably intense environment every day, but generally, once recovered from surgery, they will never see the patient again. In cardiology, a person may have a heart attack, they have treatment and go on with life. I have a colleague who is a nurse for Parkinson's patients and even she admitted that they don't see the range of issues we do.

It's the inspiring patients that keep you going and keep you smiling. They're the ones who keep you loving what you learn every day. Like all of my colleagues, I've had patients who have endured very severe attacks and symptoms and they're so scared of the medications, let alone upscaling those treatments. They have young families and even businesses, but they've powered through. It's these everyday people who are just so brave at every step of the way. But everyone is brave in their own way, and when the people who are really struggling have a breakthrough or a little win, it is a great feeling.

And there's the ones who just smile through the tears and say they're okay with all the hard decisions we've got to make. That in fact they're more worried about family members; that if only they could absorb their family's pain and worries they would.

Determining the value of a well-placed and well-timed hug to someone with MS is something I've been working on for a long time in my mind. I think early in my career I didn't understand it. I know I certainly misjudged a few times but learned pretty quickly from those attempts! But over the years it's become more instinctual. Creating that additional personal connection is important for me. It's my way of conveying to the patient 'You got this, and I believe in you.'

***

Eat the cake, travel at every opportunity, buy the shoes!

My best advice to those newly diagnosed? That MS isn't your whole life, it is only one part of your life. It's not who you are and not what you are. Life is still about fun and enjoyment and you need to surround yourself with people who make you feel good. Eat the cake, travel at every opportunity, buy the shoes!

I think it's terribly important to work out what defines you aside from the MS. For many, they may have to relearn or revisit how they want to be seen so as the MS isn't the only thing (or maybe isn't even in the equation) of defining them as a person.

To be honest, it's only because of a personal health challenge that I've learned the brilliance of my own advice. Those particular challenges, as well as entering the world of MS nursing, solidified the 'live life to the fullest' mindset for me.

I always tell people quite openly and frequently to surround themselves with people they love and who love them back. And you've got to be able to laugh at yourself as well. And the people who get that – the people who do exactly that – are the people that I see in my clinic who do better with the disease course. They don't get hung up on every little part of the disease and how it affects them.

And you've got to be prepared to possibly lose a few friends along the way as well. When the times get tough, you will cherish the people who were there for you and just stayed normal.

***

So I started this story on a reflection that – after three decades of being a nurse – it was time for me to take time out; time for me. The realisation that I needed time out wasn't something I woke up one day and suddenly realised. Nor was it something I could implement immediately. We hear about people (even our colleagues) who literally pull stumps overnight and take a sab-batical from life. This was not my situation!

I had been at the same hospital for thirty-three years and same department for twenty-three of those years. During that time, opportunities arose and I grabbed them. One of those was the possibility to pursue further study. Undertaking a PhD in multiple sclerosis had been a dream of mine for a while, although I was pretty sure it would be impossible. But.... after more than three decades in nursing I thought I would try anyway. Initially I was accepted for master's research at the University of Notre Dame in Sydney and eventually allowed to progress onto a doctorate due to my strong results. I was elated!

That elation turned a little to despair when the reality of exhausting, full time work, the long commute back and forth and conducting part-time PhD research hit. On top of this I had a new house with a matching mortgage that was through the roof and given that I was a person who enjoyed (and probably needed) a social life as well, it was only a matter of time before all the worlds collided. And collide they did big time; the battle was on! Yet I was too stubborn to make changes.

Soon into my doctoral research another quandary came and simply knocked my socks off.

A seemingly innocent visit to my GP to address my constant tiredness led to tests and a diagnosis of disseminated thyroid cancer.

To short-cut the story, I found myself in quagmire of shock, surgeries and having to slow down. Despite promising myself I would heed the warning and finally slow down, my first set of follow up results from the surgery and treatment were less than promising and I found myself yet again in the quagmire of shock, surgery and wrapping my brain around how to slow down even more.

I really have no clue how I got through 2016, but I did. My much awaited and planned for fiftieth birthday party needed to be cancelled when I was still too unwell to deal with it. It was eventually rescheduled for two months later, at which point I had decided to tell the cancer to go to hell and stay there! I adored my party; I laughed and cried and danced and sang and cher-ished every minute with my loved ones.

Meanwhile, I had resumed work as well: I was still in charge of a thriving and chaotic workplace, albeit one with disappearing funding that necessitated us stretching every minute from every day. My voluntary duties with the MSNA and MS Nurses International Certification Board also continued to provide huge satisfaction and certainly great results but not without me contributing a great amount of time and effort as well.

So yet again I find myself wondering how I'm back despairing the declining time I have to spend on the things that truly made me buoyant. In my heart I wished I could spend all my time on the research project and just get away. I adored the doctoral research and suddenly started to resent my need to work. Those feelings just crept up bit by bit, but still this ashamed me. To be completely honest, I felt ashamed of myself for feeling this way. And that's not me.

In an amalgam of irony and self-doubt, I was then confronted with two big awards in 2016, which totally and utterly blew me away. Feelings of inadequacy and unworthiness overtake any possible joy in receiving these accolades. The first award was the ubiquitous June Halper Award, which was presented in Washington, USA in May that year. The June Halper Award for Excellence in MS Nursing represents leadership and creativity in the care of people with MS and their families. The award signifies an energy of purpose to provide the most up-to-date comprehensive care possible. This was only the second time in its twenty-year history that it had been awarded to a MS Nurse leader outside of North America. In time, I got over myself and warmly grew to love the June Halper Award and all that it meant, mostly because of my love and respect for June. To be honest, it's now one of my most treasured things.

I could not seem to escape the feelings of how significantly this recognition of my career achievements distressed me. However, I learnt from that experience and was then able to accept, with considerably more grace, the MS Australia John Studdy award when announced later in November of that year. The John Studdy Award is MS Australia's highest honour and is awarded annually to individuals who have made a significant contribution to the MS movement and community in Australia. I must have recovered from my distress to some degree and the MS Australia awarding committee reflected that my speech touched their hearts. If only I could just remember what I said....

To cap off the year, my husband was then presented with an opportunity to head up his business in China and move to Shanghai. Seriously? China? No way! I had never been there, but I argued with Troy that I didn't need to. I was certain that it was a filthy and backward country and there wasn't the slightest possibility that I could leave my friends, my family and my children in Australia. Somehow, he convinced me to at least travel over and take a look before dismissing the opportunity altogether.

I just wanted to get the trip done with so we could say no and move on.

What I discovered in Shanghai was a vibrant, alive and very-much westernised city. It wasn't filthy, as I had expected, and in fact it was sort of pretty groovy. The year ended with us saying yes to the opportunity and jumping up and down a little...well, a lot!

My wish to get off the hamster wheel could possibly come true without the need to disappoint anyone! I could leave and go with him and given that I was almost at the write up stage for my PhD, I could write and write and not work for the first time since age 12! Could this really be true?

Contemplating and then facilitating a change that big was overwhelming, but I knew inherently the move overseas gave me the opportunity to rest. I looked at this next phase as a way of dealing with my 'fixing it fatigue.' I'd recognised for some time that I was experiencing a form of compassion fatigue (which I'd far rather call 'fixing it fatigue' because the thought of besmirching the sentiment of compassion is too damaging to me) but I was so caught up in it that I don't think I would have been able to let go of everything voluntarily. So, in that sense, the move overseas was a gift. I would have kept holding on to everything – for lots of reasons – even though I fundamentally knew it wasn't good for me; and also not good for the people around me.

But that's part of compassion/fixing it fatigue. You can't always see the forest for the trees. It's easier to avoid change than to confront it.

And the move overseas also allowed me to walk away with all of my dignity and grace intact; I wasn't leaving my clinic or my colleagues to go to another organisation or clinic. There'd been many times where working at a clinic or hospital closer to home would have made better sense, but I was invested in Westmead – on many levels. So while closing the door on this phase of my career was a lot to process, I really believe it was done in a way that was much more acceptable to everyone. It sat much more comfortably with me that I wasn't letting anyone down for purely selfish reasons; the decision was based on my desire to be with my husband and support him, not because I wanted to move clinics, change directions or simply take a personal break.

I resigned from my workplace of thirty-three years just prior to Christmas 2016. My university supervisors were ecstatic that I could concentrate solely on my doctoral research and I was excited and at the same time a little in awe of the project ahead.

***

The value of kindness and connection. It's a two-way street.

One thing researching my PhD has taught me it that everyone has got a story about hardship or disappointment or something that shaped them prior to their diagnosis with MS. So I now channel those experiences and coach my patients that they made it through those challenges and became stronger because of it. If I can have them understand that, then I think I can convince them that they can conquer MS too. It's often a question I lead with in a session with a newly diagnosed patient – "Tell me about some hardships you've had in your life beforehand?"

And allowing me to see behind the scenes has been a gift that writing my PhD has given me. In fact, researching for my dissertation changed my nursing style in unbelievable ways. I also know that I want to work in an environment that does things a little differently with MS patients, rather than just asking when bloods are due, how treatments are going, what particular symptoms are feeling like.

I could laughingly say that I didn't realise how little I knew about MS nursing until I did my PhD. I was classified as an expert nurse, but I've come to realise I was an expert within an organisational setting that left me very little time to ask the questions that I needed to ask to be able to best understand the patient's needs better. There was only ever time to monitor the mundane life things that were required to adhere to a treatment plan. I just felt I never had time to learn a patient's personal story or understand the unique person I was treating in a way that was sensitive to them and their own needs. Basically, everyone had to fit into the organisation's treatment model, which I felt was severely lacking in a patient-centric focus.

And you have to understand that I really prided myself on working within that model for many, many years and I certainly believed in the doctors on our team, but one of the biggest things I learned in researching my PhD was that we weren't asking the important questions. The questions we led with may have been ones that were important for safety of care but the answers to those questions weren't the information the patient wanted heard. Such things as their own story, where they came from, what had previously happened, what their care had been like before, how they felt about having MS, how MS impacted themselves and their family...

And the reason these questions are so important is because when patients make the decision to accept and follow our advice, we're asking them to trust us; to trust us enormously in taking up those decisions. Yet we'd generally been making those decisions without any clue about where the patient had come from and what might be important to them.

If I knew then what I know now, I would definitely nurse in a very different way. I would listen to my intuition a lot more, I wouldn't watch the clock as much and I think I would be more assertive in guarding my nursing time and also making sure that my nursing time was really my nursing time, not a heap of admin time disguised as nursing. All of that may get me fired next week, but those ideals are what I'd would ultimately strive for.

A few of the take home points from my research, which relate specifically to nursing practices, are things that are so simple and logical yet so inestimable to achieve.

Firstly, become a more active listener. For all the reasons I've just explained, listening to establish and gain trust is so precious. When I learned to listen and not talk was when I adjusted my consultation technique. But when you've only got twenty minutes to cover thirty-two areas, your style of questioning is very different purely for survival purposes.

My second take-home point is to explore becoming a more open and loving practitioner. Nursing has evolved in the time that I've been doing it to where it's now pretty standard to show a personalised level of care for your patients but also maintain a certain distance. I think every nurse out there would understand what I mean.

But I firmly believe a well-placed pat on the shoulder or a hug when someone clearly needs it can work wonders. And nurses are really good at reading what a patient needs, they just have to be courageous enough to engage and connect with people. And as nurses we want to be engaged and connected to our patients because we want them to trust us and follow our advice, especially in those times when they're feeling vulnerable, overwhelmed and out of control. The tiniest of gestures can dramatically change the trajectory of a patient's path.

And finally, MS nurses need to take better care of themselves if they have any hope of caring for their patients adequately. The role of the MS nurse has changed so dramatically over the last fifteen years. It used to be that an enormous part of our job was giving injection training and symptomatic support to patients, which in itself is a comprehensive undertaking. But now, the job entails so many more responsibilities. The number of DMTs has increased four-fold and so too have the onerous duties to manage those treatments. We keep hearing over and over that our nursing colleagues feel like they're drowning.

For so many years I thought that caring for the patients was the only thing that mattered and I simply didn't realise the value and importance of looking after myself. It took me falling to rock bottom whilst I was researching my PhD to realise this. I was researching and writing the theme of 'Battling the Demons,' which is all about depression, anxiety and mental health. I was so bogged down in information and transcripts and the organisation of it all and I was completely overwhelmed. Finally I asked for help, which was so easily given once I asked, and frankly people were astounded I hadn't asked for help earlier because what I was undertaking was enormous. But I guess we all want to be the exception to the rule. We all have a bit of the bullet-proof hero complex in us.

I so passionately want the MS community to embrace the precious notion of finding out the patient's story. Those little acts of kindness go such a long way in getting the patient to accept the care we're offering. It sounds so simple but I can't emphasise how important it is.

The value of kindness and connection. It's a two-way street. The patient benefits but it also enhances our professional experience and fulfilment. And that in itself is a form of self-care.

My own MS nursing journey to date has been one of serendipity, survival, self-doubt to self-reliance and steadfast compassion. And yet I still feel the best is yet to some. With all my heart, I hope the global MS nursing community recognise the extent and enormity of the leadership role they play. I think sharing our stories, even the non-perfect parts (especially these!), enables us to process all we deal with better. And that can only be a good thing. We see so much mental and physical suffering, but also much inspiration and hope. It really is an amazing, wonderful, priceless role. I am truly grateful every day.

My hopes for the future treatment and management of MS:

A cure is why we're all here. We never give up hope that there is going to be a cure. I felt so lucky to work with scientists alongside our clinic at Westmead Hospital and those scientists working in the field of MS actually predated our MS clinic. So when they say 'we will have a cure,' I unequivocally believe them and I also believe we're moving faster towards a cure then we ever have before. It's only going to get better and better.

It causes me sadness though, because I know there's going to be a lot of people who aren't going to benefit from a cure when we do crack it. But I have to hold faith that it is still going to be a tremendous thing for the future.

I only have to think about what the development of monoclonal antibodies has done in the fight to stop relapses of MS (treatments such as Lemtrada and Tysabri) and those treatments have changed lives. I've been practicing as a MS nurse and involved in the clinical trials of these treatments in Australia from the beginning, so to see what they're doing in terms of stopping relapses is incredible. I compare my patients who joined the clinical trials of these monoclonal antibody DMTs and it is mind blowing to see how they're thriving.

When I first started in the clinic, we would have had five or six people a week who needed to have an infusion of methyl prednisolone to halt a relapse. Now, across the hundreds and hundreds of patients we saw at the clinic, we'd be lucky to have one every month.

So quite simply, my holy grail is something that will cure MS and won't have serious side effects. And to be honest, I don't think some neurologists understand the impact and price that many patients pay in poor mental health whilst being on some of the medications with potentially life-threatening side effects. It weighs very heavily on some of them.

And of course, there's the damage caused by MS in the interim between having attacks and getting onto a treatment. Are we ever going to be able to repair that? My hope is also yes.

My advice for nurses beginning their career:

•   For nurses beginning their career in the field, I can't urge you enough to find your support network. Not necessarily only MS nurses, but anyone in the profession you think will be able to provide that grounding effect. Make sure you can relate to them and the work they do and you're comfortable talking to them.

•   Work out what you need to do to be able to protect yourself in this occupation, very much the same way that you would try to teach patients to do so in their own lives.

•   Prioritise looking after yourself and pay great attention to it. For me, it was about ensuring I had time out from the job, about making sure I spent my down time not working, about deciding not to check emails as soon as I got home at night. Exercise remains my linchpin. If I stop exercising, then I know everything else is going to go south. And obviously choosing to eat well, sleep well and say no to things that add to your workload without enriching your life.

•   Make sure your home life is balanced, so that you can aim for a good balance between home and work and that both are providing you with joy and relief and stimulation.

•   Make sure you plan ahead for time out.

•   Try to schedule a non-clinical day at least once a week so you can stay on top of your admin and remain organised.

•   Through writing my PhD I came to realise the most patients simply wanted to be cared for. They didn't necessarily expect you to fix or solve every problem. They just wanted to be heard and cared for. And when you remove that pressure of having to fix each and every item – many of which are simply out of your control – then you will have more time and energy to care for the person in front of you.

- And don't be afraid to push back if you're being asked to do too much and it's effecting your physical or mental health. There's no embarrassment simply saying, 'I can't do this.' In fact, I wish I'd done more of that before it was too late.

- And finally, appreciate your colleagues and your nursing friends and all their different points of view. To start each day with a purposeful and positive intention and affirmation. This helps to shape the day and provide you with some respite during the tough times. Fill your tank first and then you can get on with the joyous business of filling everyone else's too!

MEGAN WEIGEL
Jacksonville Beach, Florida, United States of America

"Be who god meant for you to be and you will set the world on fire."
- St Catherine of Siena.

....

I was born in Maryland, just outside of Washington DC but I was kind of a sick little kid growing up. I suffered through a lot of sinus-type issues and then the ensuing surgeries to alleviate that. The surgeries and sickness meant I was often out of school for long periods of time during my early adolescence. I guess I was lucky I was a self-driven kid because it actually meant I did okay at school despite everything else. But I really think that interaction with the medical world from an early age shaped my future career path tremendously.

Many years later when I was deciding what to study at college, I figured that medical school would be the most obvious choice for me. However, deep down I knew I wasn't one hundred percent sure... maybe, instead, physical therapy was the right thing for me? This was back in 1993 and the field of physical therapy was booming. I worked my way through a volunteer stint over the summer vacation to road test the field, only proving that it wasn't the right fit for me after all.

Around this time, I was also taking calculus at college and found myself really struggling with it. Actually, I hated it! I realised that unless I had significant tutoring in the subject, I probably wasn't going to make it through medical school. Coincidentally, my aunt was going through graduate school to become a certified nurse anaesthetist and it dawned on me how cool that sounded! Becoming a nurse practitioner also meant I wouldn't be in school as long and could get out into the world and practice sooner. It really was a career move that was right up my alley.

I gained entrance to and graduated from the University of Florida's nursing program, then moved to California for a year before returning to Florida to complete my Masters. I never planned to stay in Florida, but despite that, I've lived in Florida longer than I ever lived in Maryland where I grew up.

Clearly I've always been science-minded but not necessarily mathematically inclined. At the same time, I'm also a fairly creative person and I felt that once I was in nursing school and learning about the philosophy of caring there would be room to continue to be creative in the midst of all the science. From an early age, I knew I was a deeply empathetic being and think I'm pretty in touch with people. When I put all these characteristics together, a career in nursing just fit for me from the get go.

I began my career as a nurse practitioner in a neurology clinic in 2001. And to be honest, those early days were scary. I was only a few years into my nursing certification and I felt like I knew nothing about the neurology field! In America, we were only given about two minutes of training on multiple sclerosis during under-grad study, which then expanded into about four minutes during my master's programme! Can I tell you something really horrifying? For many years I thought MS (multiple sclerosis) was like MD (muscular dystrophy) and I had a master's degree in nursing! As embarrassing as this admission is, it just goes to illustrate how little specialised training our degrees gave us at the time.

And this varies from country to country. Some countries – such as the United Kingdom – have placed a major emphasis on the role of the MS nurse and offer dedicated streams of training for MS within their nursing schools. Due to the burden of MS on the UK's health system, the MS nurse's programme is now a very well-recognised field.

Luckily, I was mentored by an amazing nurse, Tina Butterfield, who introduced me to people living with MS. Bit by bit the fear started to subside and curiosity took over as I found my feet. My board certification is "Family Nurse Practitioner," and MS is a condition that affects the whole family. Very quickly I came to enjoy the aspects of my role that involved patient education, and I fell in love with the science behind multiple sclerosis and the care involved for people living with MS and their families.

This first position in the neurology practice – combined with mentoring that really resonated with me – gave me a little bit of time to build up my exposure to MS. In those early days in neurology I would work nine- and ten-hour days. I could easily spend my working day at the clinic and then come home after my shift and continue with further reading because I was so fascinated with the science, but I was also focussed on refining my instincts when it came to treating patients and their families. I loved it so much that I kept this routine going for many years; the long days just didn't faze me whilst I was so wrapped up accelerating my skills and knowledge base.

I became more and more familiar with the myriad of ways the disease could present in people; and the more people I saw the greater I trusted my intuition. This was particularly helpful in trying to interpret how many MS events a patient may have experienced so that we could gain more clarity in determining treatment options.

Instincts and disease course familiarity are certainly important at any stage of a nurse's career, but some twenty years ago, when I first started out, what we knew about MS was somewhat different to the vast amount of information we have now. No truer is that fact when it comes to diagnostic processes. We were in that transition phase between the Schumacher, Poser and McDonald criteria, where we would often have to hold back for a patient's exacerbations to reveal themselves further whilst we decoded and interpreted those events before pronouncing an official diagnosis of MS.

The McDonald criteria, which were developed in 2001 by an international expert panel and have since been revised several times, provide recommendations on the diagnosis of MS. The criteria consist of a combination of clinical, imaging, and paraclinical tests and were intended to replace the Poser criteria and the older Schumacher criteria.

In very simplified terms, the diagnosis of multiple sclerosis can be made if there is fulfilment of criteria involving number of relapses, MRI lesions, spinal fluid findings, and/or progression of disability.

The criteria are named after Ian McDonald (1933-2006), a New Zealand neurologist, who devised the original criteria with his international colleagues in 2001.

Multiple sclerosis can be difficult to diagnose because there is no single test that can determine a person has MS. The process of diagnosis involves obtaining evidence from a clinical examination, medical history, lab tests and MRI imaging of the brain and sometimes the spinal cord. These tests are intended to rule out other possible causes of a person's neurological symptoms and to gather data consistent with the diagnosis of MS.

A key principle for diagnosing MS is to uncover evidence that demonstrates lesions in the central nervous system (brain and spinal cord) showing DIS, or 'dissemination in space' and DIT - 'dissemination in time.' DIS suggests that damage has occurred in more than one place in the nervous system and DIT denotes that damage has occurred more than once.

New research evidence and evolving knowledge since the original 2001 McDonald Criteria for diagnosing MS compelled a 30-member international panel of MS experts to consider whether revisions would improve the speed and accuracy of the diagnosis of MS while reducing the possibility of misdiagnosis. The result of the criteria's 2017 review was a revision to the criteria, which enabled neurologists to determine a diagnosis after a single MS event.

***

I didn't know anyone living with multiple sclerosis when I made the decision to pursue a career as a MS nurse practitioner. But I think because of the sheer volume of information I was taking on board and the way I was immersing myself in the job and patient education, I started meeting many other people in the field: Nurses, physicians, rehab professionals, non-profit champions.... and the list goes on. It didn't take me long to realise that I had found myself in a really special place. I was overwhelmed by the altruism in MS care, as well as the collaboration across specialties, which is not present in most branches of medicine.

But my first truly personal connection to MS was a chance meeting within the first year of my nursing practice, when I had met a woman who had graduated from college at a similar time to me. We were both the same age, both ended up practicing in neurology and we both met at a workshop for one of the large MS pharmaceutical companies. It was 2001 and coincidentally the first pharma conference either of us had attended. And those were the days where the big pharma companies would fly you to exotic locations and put everything on for you!

We struck up an easy friendship after discovering so many similarities in our lives. Some years later she was travelling back from an overseas vacation and her hands went numb during the flight. She immediately put it down to a lack of circulation whilst flying but when sensation failed to return after several days, she consulted the neurologist she worked with. He immediately referred her for an MRI and very quickly they confirmed she had MS.

To this day, I still find it quite eerie that we both travelled along such similar paths in starting our nursing studies at the same time, we then met at a MS conference and both worked in the field of MS. How was it that someone – for all intents and purposes – was exactly like me but found herself being diagnosed with multiple sclerosis? Subsequently, she left neurology a few years after her diagnosis and went into the field of pain management before returning to neurology several years ago and finding a good fit for herself in MS care. She is truly able to empathise with those living with MS and provide an incredible level of care. She is also a tireless advocate for her patients and herself.

She's one of the best nurse practitioners I know in MS and she has a pretty amazing story. I definitely think it gives her a unique insight into her patients. She will divulge her diagnosis when relevant, but she doesn't broadcast that she is living with MS. I know of a few other health care professionals that are very active in the MS arena, either as nurse practitioners or working for pharmaceutical companies and they too have MS. It's an interesting dynamic to be practicing in the field of a condition you have been diagnosed with. I often wonder how you would strike a balance between living with and managing a condition that you also have to work in each day?

***

I think creativity is a wonderful skill to have in nursing and I would hope other nurses have similar characteristics. It can be a real bonus – particularly in a hospital environment – to be able to manipulate the resources in a creative way. Come to think about it, I believe that nursing is all about creativity; we run the risk of being stuck under an avalanche of paperwork at times and to exercise our creativity through patient management is a good offset to the minutia of administrative work.

And creativity can alleviate the challenges we face in treating patients. Nearly every challenge we encounter will fall in one of two areas; either system-based challenges or patient-based challenges.

I almost feel as if there's a bit more control over the system-based challenges, despite the fact that you rarely actually have control! A common example of this are the many challenges we confront getting patients onto disease modifying therapies (DMTs). To be honest, I've had to learn how to play the game when it comes to dealing with either our health system in America or the pharmaceutical companies so as I can get my patient onto what we believe is the best DMT for them, faster. Despite knowing how the game is played and when to play it, it's still tremendously frustrating.

Even the seemingly simple task of scheduling MRIs for patients can turn into a massive process; the time it takes just seems so ridiculously wasted. It can take multiple calls and twenty minutes to get a basic request approved for an MRI for a patient who has had MS for over a decade. To me, there's no reason why there should be a big discussion about an approval of this nature and twenty minutes here and there may not seem like a lot, but it all adds up.

Then of course in America, we also have the extra layer of administration to deal with for insurance companies or the Medicare/Medicaid system. Every state has different commercial and government insurance plans with different formularies for drugs. In other instances, people may qualify for subsidised treatments and DMT's but then the funding for those may dry up. I see plenty of cases where someone will have access to subsidised drugs for three or so months and then suddenly the grant funding will terminate. It's so frustrating and stressful for all involved.

To add another layer of complexity, in Florida, we have a large active duty military and Veterans, so naturally, we also have to be highly familiar with their insurance and medical system, which is different yet again to everything else.

All-in-all there's times when continuity of care across the board can be tough. And unfortunately, the funding games in particular are the ones you can't win.

The challenges I see that are patient-based are the cases when the patient is so very unwell, not necessarily from MS symptoms, but instead from an unhealthy lifestyle. Situations where poor lifestyle choices lead to obesity, depression, high blood pressure, or diabetes. And because they have MS, they feel disempowered. So they go into a bit of a spiral and develop all these other lifestyle complications, which are really going to be the things that affect them – and their MS – more so than anything else.

Trying to help my patients and their families understand that a healthier way of living is available, enjoyable and will certainly result in a happier day for them is inevitably challenging. And whilst I might be able to play games with the health system for the benefit of the patient, I can't – and would never – play games with human beings.

All in all, the most frustrating thing about my job is really when I see a person living with MS that I know can live a better life, and whether it's their own nature or my technique or the inability to relate to them, but I can't get them to buy into the culture of making positive lifestyle modifications.

Have I ever been in a situation I didn't know how to fix? Oh goodness yes! Every. Single. Day. Or at least it feels like it! There are those times when you will devote so much energy crafting and personalising resources for patients to help them live as healthier humans and in turn, manage their MS symptoms better. Yet deep down you know that they're going to leave your office and disregard all of the advice despite the fact that ten minutes prior they were vigorously nodding and agreeing with your suggestions, purely to keep you happy. Or maybe it all just seemed so much easier with you cheerleading…and harder for the patient if you are not in front of them. There's so much psychology that goes into a person reaching a decision to make a change. And sometimes, it's just not the time for them. Sometimes, it requires three or ten more visits. And that's okay, but for a person who puts her heart into her work, it can lead to a depletion of personal resources.

Also, some of our more progressed patients – and I see this predominantly in men – are finding themselves in a situation where it's becoming harder and harder for their family to care for them. I see the families losing not only their energy but losing their hope. In those situations, it breaks me to say there is truly not much to offer besides support. I feel this happening maybe twice a week. That's really hard….. that's really very hard for me. I suspect I feel it harder than the patient does because I blame myself that there's little I can do, whereas the families are often in a phase of dulled acceptance.

The number of DMTs that are now available to treat MS has been the most significant advance during my career. Whilst the advancements in the efficacy of the DMTs are impressive – and keeping in mind that nobody has studied all thirteen of them head-to-head so we don't really know unequivocally if one is better than the other – but I'm most excited that our patients have more choices now. And those choices open up more possibilities for a disease that can seem pretty hopeless and also allow the patient to feel like they can retain some control, at least through their choice of treatments. We didn't have this luxury of choice before.

The other promising change I'm seeing in the United States is the recognition of the value of integrated care. We now have MS centres that are providing a tremendously positive impact for the care in MS.

An integrative and holistic approach in treatment has always been personally important to me and I see it being embraced by so many other MS nurses as well. Promoting the importance of exercise and nutrition to live as a healthy human is nothing new but it's only been in the last few years that we now have data to back this up in terms of treating MS. In particular, over the last decade we've seen a great deal reported about the benefits of exercise and modalities such as yoga and Pilates as proven methods for rehabilitation.

And the benefits of exercise for people living with MS are huge. What is ironic is that whilst we've been promoting exercise for better patient health for a long time, it's only now that we are seeing more research data reported that exercise is becoming 'medically' accepted if you will. In nursing we know what we know, but in a traditional medical sense, the hard research was required for the doctors and patients alike to fully get on board!

We have several support groups in my area for people living with MS. Each are different and will naturally attract people at various points of their journey with MS, thus forming the character of those groups. The groups I see as providing the most uplifting experiences are those that incorporate exercise into their programme. The anecdotal feedback I receive from participants is that it changes their mindset. I've seen patients go from self-isolating and generally housebound to becoming some of the most socially active people in the community, all because of the positive effects that exercise has on a person's self-confidence. I see better bonds and support forming through these groups and the knock-on effect is a minimisation of stress and burden on their families, along with the obvious health benefits.

***

The Plot Twist... "What if I fall?"
"Oh but my darling... what if you fly?"
– Erin Hanson

One of the pivotal moments in my career was when I found myself in teacher training for yoga in early 2012. It truly was a divine inter-vention. I never wanted to be a yoga teacher; I was just doing the training to deepen my foundation of yoga. But during that course I promised myself that if I did in fact ever start teaching, I wanted it to be a programme specifically designed for people living with MS.

And this yoga training was really the beginning of self-healing for me. It was the beginning of me taking a good hard look at the story I'd been writing and carrying around about my own life.

My grandmother and stepfather had not long passed away and I was also coming to terms with my divorce. At the time, I didn't know much about healing and self-acceptance. I only knew how to do dramatic things to justify situations. This was my chance to decide whether I was going to let my story write itself or whether I was going to take the pen in my own hand.

And on paper I was on a stellar career trajectory but to be honest, I never really found my True North until I introduced yoga into my profession. To explain this, most of the people I was teaching yoga to were also my patients. So I knew what these beautiful, brave people looked like in the exam room. I knew how they could move their legs or whether they could and couldn't walk; but when we did yoga there was no correlation what-so-ever between their practice of breath and movement and their neurological examination findings.

Coincidentally around this time I discovered the work of poet Erin Hanson. She has a quote that I could never get out of my mind. "What if I fall?" "Oh but my darling... what if you fly?" I had a finite sense that there was something bigger than me involved in healing. For a long time, it was actually too scary to say out loud because after twenty years, I wondered where it was going to take my professional career? I was certainly feeling the part of Hanson's quote where you wonder "what if I fall?"

A year after completing my yoga teacher training and together with my dear friend who has MS, we founded oMS Yoga to bring free yoga classes to people living with MS. Within four years we expanded from Florida into South Carolina and Philadelphia as well. Teaching yoga made me realise that there is much more to improving the quality of life of people living with the disease than prescribing medication. And quite joyfully, teaching yoga eventually led me to my studies in integrative medicine and it has fundamentally changed the way I practice nursing and patient care every day.

But now, within such a short time, we have physicians (those who were initially so very resistant to our less traditional models of care and support) asking for our MS yoga classes. Those who were somewhat critical of yoga for MS are now seeing the benefits and improvements in their patients who take our programmes. And whilst the doctors and neurologists may be a little late to the party, it's been my experience that most MS nurses subscribe to an ethos of having the mind, body and spirit aligned to achieve the healthiest lifestyle possible.

When I first began studying yoga so as I could develop and teach classes to people with MS, I was often queried by neurologists as to when I was 'really' going to study or publish something about yoga in the clinical sense? The inference being that what I was doing with yoga and MS wasn't exactly legit until I put some hard-core research around it. Sometimes I would answer that I was too busy, but mostly I would just look at them and say, "you know, I just haven't figured out a great way to measure joy." Since they didn't know how, either, they were usually quiet.

And it was the experience of joy that made sense to me in the treatment process. Joy changes people. It heals people. And certainly, as joy began to take a greater root in my life, it began to take a greater root in my professional life. But more about my own little plot twist later.....

***

Instil hope and empowerment early...but manage expectations.

The two most common questions I'm asked by a newly diagnosed patient are 'am I going to have a normal life?' and 'am I going to be able to continue working?'

'Can I have a normal life?' Wow... That's a really big open-ended question and the answer will be different for everyone that asks. I guess I try to read the person to understand whether they're a naturally optimistic person or rather a pessimistic one? Maybe even if they have a spiritual belief system? And I go from there...

I really believe that if you instil hope and empower a person early, then they will do better no matter what they're facing. They handle things better from the beginning; they handle adversity better and they adapt better. I've been a MS nurse a little over fifteen years and I'd still consider myself a newbie compared with many of my colleagues, but I know that the face of MS has changed so much, just in that short time, that the expanse of hope has only grown larger.

No matter what stage of the disease people and their families are experiencing, one of the other most common questions I'm asked is about new therapies and whether or not the disease or the damage can be reversed?

Discussing disease or symptom reversal can be a hard thing to explain to patients because ultimately you want to give people the words they want to hear; you want to be positive and hopeful. And with some of our newer therapies and with others in the pipeline, we're starting to see stability of disease in populations of people where we were not previously seeing such things. To me, that's very significant and adds hope and positivity.

So I think pointing out that some people now stabilise on the newer DMTs, rather than continue to progress, (or progress much more slowly), is such a positive outcome that we couldn't achieve when I started in MS.

The hardest cases I experience are the people who have more

advanced MS and scramble for treatments that might not be the best for them. These patients seek treatments in clinics by practitioners that haven't performed the clinical trials or they undertake modalities that have no scientific basis. And these treatments are generally prohibitively expensive and then that cost just adds to the burden. I literally cry when I hear about my patients putting themselves through such things. They do it because they're so desperate and whilst I've never been in their shoes, I can imagine the various things that drive them to the point of seeking out treatments and advice that – from a clinical perspective – we know is probably ineffective and potentially harmful.

It's a difficult and cruel conversation to have with someone who is experiencing progressing symptoms and also advancing in their disease course because we do not have as many treatment options. It's also compounded by the fact that we know that people are generally faring better if they are able to start on a DMT earlier into their diagnosis, and some of these folks were diagnosed decades before the first DMT. Fortunately, we do have one treatment for primary progressive MS, as well as a new DMT that was studied in an active secondary progressive group. A clinician just needs to consider that the person for whom they are considering a specific DMT looks somewhat like that clinical trial population.

Managing patient expectations is a constantly changing battle field and if I ever have a bad day at work, it's often because I feel I haven't managed my patient's expectations well. Or somebody felt left out or left behind... And that sometimes goes back to the people who aren't willing to change their lifestyle to feel better or are more willing to just accept an early defeat. MS is hard. I always hope with time I can change their minds.

***

Finding your True North alignment,
even amongst those crazy-eye days.

I'll be honest: It can be hard to make sure the stress of the job doesn't build up. I pray. A lot. I'm constantly reminding myself to breathe deeply. In fact, I do it all day long unbeknownst to anyone around me.

And since starting on my own journey with yoga, I've really found great benefit from the practice of breathing and mindfulness, especially amidst those chaotic days. There will be times I might feel quite unsettled during a consultation with a patient – largely due to competing attentions or previous stressors – so I'll pretend I don't have shoes on and just press my feet to the floor and find what I call my own 'true north' alignment. It's just a small move, where I'll realign my posture, take a few deep breaths, roll my shoulders back and I know the person sitting across from me has no clue what I'm doing. It's like hitting an internal re-set button. At its very root, I'm just practicing mindfulness and the habit has assisted me tremendously.

I've recently completed a fellowship in integrative medicine and one of the most fascinating concepts I've discovered is the ritual of medicine; it's a practice that has helped me tremendously. New studies are being undertaken at places like Stanford and Harvard that show great benefit to the simple performance of medical ritual and bedside manner.

Medical rituals, like religious rituals, serve to alter the meaning of an experience by naming and encompassing some of those unknown elements of that medical experience and by enabling the patient's belief in a treatment and their expectancy of healing from that treatment.

In fact, Harvard Medical School's Programs in Placebo Studies (PiPS) believes that the medical rituals are in fact critical elements necessary to mobilise the potent placebo effects. They say "For many years, the placebo effect was considered to be no more than a nuisance variable that needed to be controlled in clinical trials. Only recently have researchers redefined it as the key to understanding the healing that arises from medical ritual, the context of treatment, the patient-provider relationship and the power of imagination, trust and hope."

And whilst the PiPS research is ongoing, other proponents discuss topics such as how the medical fraternity have the capacity to generate significant feelings of hope and hence healing, which are often overlooked in our technology-obsessed health care systems.

A 2015 article in the New England Journal of Medicine (NEJM) calls these rituals "therapeutic encounter." The NEJM article explains:

"In a broad sense, placebo effects are improvements in patients' symptoms that are attributable to their participation in the therapeutic encounter, with its rituals, symbols, and interactions. These effects are distinct from those of discrete therapies and are precipitated by the contextual or environmental cues that surround medical interventions, both those that are fake and lacking in inherent therapeutic power and those with demonstrated efficacy. This diverse collection of signs and behaviors includes identifiable health care paraphernalia and settings, emotional and cognitive engagement with clinicians, empathic and intimate witnessing, and the laying on of hands."

A related idea was proposed by Psychology Professors Art Bohart and Karen Tallman in their 1999 book How Clients Make Therapy Work, in which they say that for most issues, the efficacy of mental health treatments come not from the particular approach that the therapist uses but whether or not the patient and therapist establish a meaningful connection. If they do, therapy is more likely to be effective across most measures – if they don't, nothing done in therapy is likely to help much.

Whilst the notion of the ritual of medicine might be a little flaky for the more traditionally inclined, Dr. Abraham Verghese, a notable three-time best-selling author and professor of Theory and Practice of Medicine and Associate Chair of Internal Medicine at Stanford University was awarded the National Humanities Medal In 2015 for his research in the area.

In a well-recognised speech to medical school graduates from Stanford's esteemed school of medicine, he says "You are also participating in a timeless ritual ... when you get to examine a patient. You are in a ceremonial white gown. They are in a ceremonial paper gown. You stand there not as yourself, but as the doctor. As part of that ritual they will allow you the privilege of touching their body, something that in any other walk of life would be considered assault.

"The ritual properly performed earns you a bond with the patient... The ritual is timeless, and it matters. People take care of other people."

Dr. Verghese keeps framed in his bedroom a quote from a 16th-century physician named Paracelsus: "This is my vow: to love the sick, each and all of them, more than if my own body were at stake." This statement alone embodies the spirit of the ritual of medicine.

And of course, the flipside to looking after your patients is being able to look after yourself. In that way, exercise has been a great saviour for me. Every night when I leave the office I try to take a walk or make time for a yoga class so that I can better manage my stress.

Stress and burn out is certainly endemic in nursing and I daresay more so in nurses working in the field of chronic conditions, especially where people don't tend to improve. It can be a disheartening burden to take on and I see the stress manifesting when the nurses become ill themselves. And of course there are those days – all too frequent – where you can look at your colleagues and just see the crazy in their eyes; and that's when we've all got to look after each other and nudge a gentle reminder to chill out.

It's an issue we openly discuss at our association meetings as we work out ways to reign each other in and to find that buddy or mentoring system to care for each other. The big problem is that we're universally here because we love what we do and for the most part we all have the same personality traits that lead us down the same path and cause us to just keep on going. Let's just liken it to the blind leading the blind! It's actually a little weird to stop and consider how we look after ourselves, because we're there to look after our patients, first and foremost.

But the 'crazy eye' days are far outnumbered by the really great days. I get to meet so many inspiring people and their families, who just have such amazing spirit and a determined will; I'm constantly uplifted by the prevailing human spirit in our MS community. One woman I know has been living with MS for some decades now. She uses a motorised wheel chair to get around and it is operated through a straw mechanism, but I never ever see her without a smile on her face. In fact, I remember that about six years ago, she organised to go tandem sky diving whilst she still had some use of her arms remaining. It's the spirit of those people that I always keep in my pocket to get me through the crazy eye days.

There are so many people who have said that the diagnosis of multiple sclerosis changed their life for the better. Those are the people who realised they weren't really living before the diagnosis and that MS has given them a new perspective and better priorities in life. And those are the people who then go on to teach others so much.

The best advice I'd like to offer to someone newly diagnosed with MS is along the same lines as the advice I'd give to my own colleagues; if you don't have alignment in your life then it's all just going to be more difficult from the get go. In simple terms, if your mind and spirit are out of balance, then your body certainly will be too. I so often find that a newly diagnosed person will have an innate sense of what needs to be the most meaningful priority in their life from that point forward, so for a MS nurse to help them articulate that priority and keep it at the forefront of their mind is really an important part of our job. Especially in the beginning of the diagnosis, it's just a big scary spiral. I often compare it to a necklace that you can't untangle. Like, what do you do first? That's why helping patients to stick to their priorities is an important part of this puzzle. It can provide clarity and direction for a patient.

***

"Be who god meant for you to be and you will set the world on fire."
- St Catherine of Siena

The plot twist I alluded to earlier had been percolating away as a slow burn for some time. Then out of the blue it reached boiling point and just hit me.

I continued to passionately devote a lot of time to the Florida chapter of the National MS Society as both a member of the Health-care Advisory Committee and a Research Advocate, as well as serving on the editorial board of the International Journal of MS Care. I had become a member of the International Organisation of MS Nurses (IOMSN) many years prior and was now stepping into leadership and executive board roles there. This culminated in being elected as president of the organisation around this time and also garnering the accolade of being one of North Florida's 'Top 100 Nurses.' I was so grateful at how full and rewarding my career had become.

And working at the neurology clinic continued to be wonderful. I was in a great environment with a great team, but I now knew without a shadow of doubt that there was something bigger and better that all my patients could do other than just take the prescribed DMT. Prescriptions and medicine work, but I don't believe that medicine has its full chance to truly work unless you allow the healing in and you allow all the other medicines to do their work too. Things such as spiritual medicine, nutritional medicine, breathing as medicine, movement as medicine. I began to find it harder and harder to have enough time to communicate to people exactly what I thought might be healing for them.

At the same time, I was also finding it more and more difficult to explain to my colleagues that I kind of knew that my patients were going to experience other co-morbidities because they were just going full speed ahead without rest, or ignoring past trauma without resolution to name just a few things. In my mind there was no option except that these people would become sicker and I felt my colleagues couldn't necessarily see or agree with that.

For a number of reasons I suddenly found myself at a crossroad in life about six years ago and decided to take myself off to Costa Rica for five days. It was just the tonic I needed and I returned to work feeling very brave and focused. But then another year went by and I continued to be that busy person on the hamster wheel and bit by bit I recognised that I was right back in that uncomfortable space again; I knew that my heart was not in the right place.

I remember the exact moment I woke up with a paralyzing and

consuming tightness in my chest and I just knew I had to change something before something changed me for the worse. I knew this would turn into a health crisis if I didn't, like the ones I could see would happen to my patients.

Only after I explained I was willing to risk my job on it, did my boss very begrudgingly let me take a leave of absence for a month so I could take time out to figure out what my story needed to be going forward. I happily made arrangements for my month-long sabbatical in Hawaii but just two weeks before I was to leave I found a lump in my breast. I was scared but strangely resigned about the fact at the same time. I knew this is exactly what happens when you don't heed the warnings that your body gives you. These things manifest in sickness.

Anyway, I went for my ultrasound and then a diagnostic mammogram and in my head I'm turning my month in Hawaii into a month of getting a mastectomy and undergoing chemo and radiation and then I would go back to work. In my mind, I was too late to make the fundamental changes I had dreamed of. My path was written to stay doing what I'd always done.

So to be told that I was all clear was a bit mind blowing. I knew that my story could have gone either way and I realised how very, very lucky I was. I could no longer ignore all the signs that were being put in front of me. I felt so grateful and I could only imagine that someone out there was really looking out for me and I needed to make the most of this time that I was giving myself. I simply couldn't allow myself to go away to Hawaii, only to return to the same old patterns. I had to make changes.

And indeed, big changes were afoot. I enrolled in an Integrative Medicine fellowship through the University of Arizona as soon as I returned from Hawaii and then other magical life events happened. I met a great guy, had a wonderful baby boy, and got married. All divine things that I wasn't sure would be part of my story going forward! Soon after the birth of my son, I cut back the hours I was working at the clinic and yet somehow found myself working longer hours.

Just as I was pondering how the heck less hours translated into more work, the clinic introduced a new electronic medical record (EMR) and whilst I'm pretty tech-savvy I found the EMR reducing my eye contact with my patients significantly and this didn't sit well with me at all. I estimated my interaction was reduced by some thirty percent. Up until that point the only thing keeping me alive in the clinic was the ability to establish and maintain a rapport with my patients but the moment the new EMR went in I knew I was gone. I woke up with that warning signal tightness in my stomach and gave my notice not long after, so I could set up my own practice in integrative medicine. The looks on my colleague's faces when they discovered I was leaving the neurology clinic was one of disbelief and confusion. No one could understand what I was doing...

I didn't feel particularly brave doing this. Instead I felt it was something necessary I had to do for my family, for my own life and something that I had to do for the people that I served as patients.

I often ponder how I came to be where I am now, and I keep coming back to that point in time where learning and embracing integrative medicine became fundamental to me. I inherently knew that there was so much more to offer people than merely being treated for multiple sclerosis via a 25-minute office appointment. There was just so much more I wanted to do above and beyond explaining the DMT's, pleading with people to eat healthily and stress less, hoping like heck they might even do some exercise, only to bid them farewell with an offer to see them again in three months.

So I opened my own practice with the belief in every fibre of my being that the information and research I had to give my patients on healing and managing disease couldn't be done via those traditionally short and sharp – almost rote – clinical consultations. Ultimately, I believed there was something bigger than just the tools I had learned in my traditional medical practice to heal my patients, even if a cure wasn't possible. I didn't quite have it all figured out how I'd be treating patients differently, other than just inherently knowing I had to.

About six months after graduating from my Integrative Medicine fellowship I went to sit for an exam in Advanced Practice Holistic Nursing through the American Holistic Nurses Association; I needed to prove to myself that I actually took the fellowship and practice seriously! I studied quite hard for it, as the fellowship I had just completed was actually focused around physician's training and the nursing stream was quite different. I found myself studying nursing theory for this exam and realised a lot of traditional nursing theory had origins in holistic nursing practices. I came across this 'story theory,' which essentially explains that we all have stories and they're all worth telling.

Stories are a fundamental dimension of human experience and nursing practice and story theory describes a narrative that occurs through intentional nurse to patient dialogue. Seven inquiry phases are associated with story theory, including gathering the story, reconstructing the story, connecting it to the literature, naming the complicating health challenge, describing the story plot, identifying movement toward resolving, and gathering additional stories.

From a nursing stance, you have to really pay attention to the patient's story because they lead us to the essence of the person we're treating. Through retracing all this nursing theory, it sort of hit me like a tonne of bricks that what I was so drastically missing in my own interactions with my patients was time for them to tell their story. Why hadn't I realised this before now?

So from that point on, my practice became rooted in heart-centred listening. I wanted to create a place that gave people the time – and safety – to tell their own stories. And what I've found is that the people who have followed me from my previous clinic – some of whom I've known for more than a decade – would comment 'wow... I thought you knew me, but now you REALLY know me!'

But to be honest, it's the same sentiment for me on the flip side because I don't feel crunched by time any longer and it's become so much easier to know my patients on a deeper level. My consultations now allow me to park the illness of my patients aside and explore how a person arrived at where they are and discuss the sort of life they'd like to live going forward. We then work together to author a new health narrative – achieved through a number of integrative measures – all of which will help treat their disease as well. I want to give people a platform for healing and I believe that healing begins when you're allowed to tell your story. I now have very strong convictions about this belief but strangely, I couldn't have said that a year ago.

As an important step to me gathering and reconstructing a patient's story, I spend some time in my consultations assessing what sort of trauma has been experienced throughout their life. I have to be delicate and respectful when treading through these areas but I'm seeing an undeniable pattern where a significant amount – and I mean more than eighty percent – of my patients have endured a major trauma in their life. And listening to these stories is such a difficult part of the work with my patients; I often can't fathom the amount of pain we inflict on each other as a society. But I also feel tremendously privileged to be trusted with these stories.

How many times have we witnessed or heard stories about doctors who are dismissive of ill health being caused by trauma? They may be all too quick to write off the notion of chronic health complaints that have manifested after abuse, or the loss of a loved one, or living with and through an untenable situation. They will literally close down to the idea because there's no clinical tool they can prescribe as a remedy after trauma.

To be completely honest, I probably held very similar thoughts for a while, but I now believe that what happens to our immune systems and our bodies when we're enduring chronic stress can also be a root cause of ailments. For some of my patients, a diagnosis is almost like a vindication that their stories have been heard, that living with the aftermath of trauma is a contributing factor to their ill health.

Starting my own practice has taught me how little I was able to use my skillset. It's highlighted that I could only use tiny parts of the skills I'd learned over the last twenty years. Now I feel like I can use so many more facets of the expertise I've built and that's allowed me to form much deeper relationships with my patients and also other MS nurses – mainly because I now allow myself the time! I definitely pay a lot more attention to what people tell me they believe their problems are, instead of immediately defaulting to the scientific position.

I'm so aware now that the way we practice medicine in our country strongly feeds anxiety because of the constraints and confines of our health care system. Let me give you an example: A person calls at 9am with a scary new symptom that they're feeling. Then at 1pm, they still haven't heard back from anyone about what to do or how to manage something that's really frightening them. Then at 5pm, they STILL haven't gotten a call back and the anxiety has reached fever pitch or worse still, they feel irrelevant, ignored or irrational.

Managing the issue of timeliness for follow-ups is a two-way street. I've thought about this a lot and as nurses, we have an important duty in managing the expectations of our patients in how we will manage an enquiry and ultimately follow up, but also in educating patients of the rational steps they need to take depending on whether they need advice, emergency care or something in between.

Similarly, I think we could do much more to educate our nursing community as to the impact anxiety has on exacerbating MS symptoms, which in turn impacts the outcome for the patient.

We are so time poor as nurses and time, unfortunately, is one of those resources that has become an absolute luxury, but I can't reinforce enough the importance of timely patient enquiry follow up.

I think it could be easy for us to under-estimate the debilitating anxiety that comes from living day-to-day with an unknown illness like MS. I often find it helpful to encourage our patients to ask questions and seek education so they can be better informed about MS. This may serve to eliminate some fears when they arise but may also minimise any alarm and terror people feel if they are experiencing a new or more intense symptom.

***

I hope that by telling my story I can help people living with MS and their families make a paradigm shift from thinking that they're in a hopeless situation or that their life is over, to instead believing that the diagnosis of their condition could be something they can turn around into a positive. I hope they start to ask themselves 'how can I pick myself up by the bootstraps and live perhaps in a healthier way than I would have otherwise?' Or 'how can I take this tap on the shoulder and turn it around?'

The MS nursing community, whose foundation is in the International Organization of MS Nurses, has been such an integral part of my life for nearly two decades and I'm passionate about instilling a sense of sustainable health and wellness amongst my colleagues. From time to time we've all needed someone who 'gets it' to bounce ideas around with and also to simply vent to. I talk a lot about the hope and inspiration I see in MS but there's no escaping that we also have to deal with struggles and frustrations.

And whilst our unique MS nurse community is spread throughout the world, we certainly have mighty bonds! I've formed so many wonderful connections with other MS nurses and we can all support each other in our career, our lives – really anything at all.

I'm a nurse through and through and I know I've been put here to help people heal. But I'm not always confident that I deserve to do this profession at the level I am now or that I deserve to play this intimate role in my patient's life. But I'm working on all of that and for now, I just commit to my practice and keep reminding myself that I'm here, my patient is here and that I have to believe in the relationship we've forged and that giving them anything less than every skill I have in my toolkit is a waste of their time.

To draw inspiration from Erin Hanson's quote again... "Oh but my darling... what if you fly?"

My hopes for the future treatment and management of MS:

• One thing I'd love anyone living with MS to know is just how many people are out there working for them. We have so much ground-breaking research being carried out, we know so much more than we ever did, and all this information is permeating through the advice our neurologists and MS nurses are giving back to patients. We have so many other disciplines and health care specialists working towards providing therapies and treatments and resources that will ultimately provide people living with MS and their families a healthier, happier and more fulfilling life, despite a diagnosis of MS.

• There's so much going on in the world of MS these days and I feel like it keeps increasing exponentially every year. It truly is an amazing field to be a part of and to know that you're going to help people. I can't remember who said this, but when it comes to neurological diseases, MS has the greatest number of medical advances over the last century. So that being said, anyone considering a career in the field of MS is entering at a very exciting and dynamic time.

• I believe within my life time, that if not a cure, then there will be a treatment developed that will reverse the effects of the disease. I liken it to the advances we've seen in treating HIV and AIDS. So a patient may still need to be on medication but the medication will prevent the disease from progressing and even offer disease reversal.

• I also think that we're going to start learning more about the genetics of MS and how to choose a therapy. We will see personalised medicine come to the forefront where we can choose a treatment or therapy based on the individual type of disease symptoms and progress.

- I don't subscribe to the "pharmaceutical conspiracy theory" – and yes, that's deliberately said with big quote mark around it…. I don't believe that big pharma is preventing us from finding a cure for fear of losing money in drug sales. Frankly these companies give out so much in free drug treatments that it just doesn't make sense.

My advice for nurses beginning their career:

- So the best piece of advice I could give to an MS nurse would be to maintain their own sense of well-being in order to avoid burn out. It's become a focus for me and I can't stress it enough for my colleagues and fellow practitioners. As nurses, we tend to exhibit both type A characteristics and we're people constantly on the go; and when something brings us down we run the risk of really falling hard unless we have solid wellness practices built up. If you want to have a good ride in this profession, your ticket is your own mental, physical and emotional health and well-being. Keep your car in tune!

- The importance of having a tool box of resources on hand; a 'break glass in case of emergency' sort of emergency plan is a great thing for nurses to create for their own patient management techniques but also for patients to develop for themselves.

- The importance of the timely follow up can't be underestimated.

- The importance of coordinating care. For instance, I've found it so very beneficial to just pick up the phone and coordinate with other health care specialists to follow up and explain a patient's situation rather than just assume the specialists will actually read a fax or an email.

- Really listening to what the person living with the disease believes the problem is, at that point in time. Even if you know that there's no way on earth that the problem you're addressing has been caused by what the patient is telling you, it's still a road-block the patient is feeling and it surely feeds into the illness and healing process in some way.

MICHAEL MORTENSEN
Hobart, Australia

You become a person of support for them, and they look to you to help make sense of the disease with which they live.

I grew up in north-west Victoria – right near Swan Hill – which is basically in the middle of nowhere. There wasn't a lot going on there and I only ever remember the area as being hot and flat.

It came as no surprise to anyone when I left my hometown in my late teens to move to Melbourne to find a job. I ended up working in trust and estate administration for many years and also volunteering for a number of organisations that supported adolescents and young adults living with intellectual and physical disabilities. It didn't take long for the volunteer work at The Spastic Society of Victoria and Yooralla to become a consistent part of my life but the way I found myself in those wonderful roles was quite serendipitous to say the least.

I was taking a walk on my lunch break one day and happened across an open day for volunteers. I decided to poke my head in and as I was casually browsing around and wondering what it was all about, a lady from The Spastic Society of Victoria waved and beckoned me over. "Hey, you.... come over here!" I sort of looked over both shoulders, wondering who she was yelling at and then realised it could only be me! "You'd be a perfect volunteer for us," she proclaimed. The bewildered look on my face gave her enough time to edge in and tell me all the opportunities I was about to be exposed to as a volunteer. Six years later I was still volunteering for that organisation and also support roles at Yooralla, which provides services for people with disabilities. None of this work was nursing in any form, but it was definitely granting the feeling that I was contributing in some way to someone less fortunate than myself.

But for some reason, there was always something about Tasmania that really appealed to me and I found myself constantly drawn to the notion of moving there. As much as I disliked how hot and flat Swan Hill was, perhaps returning to a rural setting was what I was seeking?

I decided to move to 'Tassie' in 1992 and where I eventually settled just outside of Hobart is the polar opposite to where I grew up. I adore living on the outskirts of a city, with only a short drive to work every day and yet returning home at night to feel like I was miles away from anything. I don't know what it is about Tasmania, but it just seems to grab hold of you. There's a beauty about the place that I haven't seen anywhere else and I've been happily living in Tassie for over 25 years now.

And for as settled as I am now, the original transition wasn't that seamless. The job in stock-broking I had accepted and was due to begin in Hobart, informed me that I'd likely have to re-locate over to Singapore within twelve months, at least if I intended to continue in the position. I hadn't moved to Tasmania to move again, so I declined the position and found myself without a job. Instead, I began work as a support worker in group homes, assisting adults living with intellectual and physical disabilities.

I dabbled away as a support worker for a while before deciding I should probably try to up-skill myself a bit more. So in my mid-30s I applied for mature-age entry to the University of Tasmania where I obtained my Bachelor of Nursing, graduating in 1998. I undertook my graduate year back in Victoria at the Alfred Hospital, specialising in infectious diseases, then transitioned to the Royal Melbourne – again in infectious diseases – for another five years, before returning to Launceston in Tasmania for two years and a position in oncology. I finally returned to Hobart where I started my nursing journey and went into the Ambulatory Care Centre (ACC) at Royal Hobart Hospital.

It was here that I developed an interest in multiple sclerosis, as this was where Tysabri infusions and IV methylprednisolone were given. In fact, I was working in the infusions suite the day we gave the first ever Tysabri infusion. We were all very intrigued by this treatment advancement and what it might do. The infusions suite was just generally a fascinating place to be as we were seeing the introduction of a lot of new treatments at this stage, not just for multiple sclerosis but also Crohns disease, rheumatoid arthritis and ankylosing spondylitis.

ACC was also the ward used by the CARE-MS study, and I was involved with the delivery of some of the first alemtuzumab infusions as part of the clinical trial. The two-year CARE-MS trial studied the efficacy and safety of alemtuzumab (Lemtrada™) as a treatment for relapsing-remitting multiple sclerosis, in comparison with subcutaneous interferon beta-1a (Rebif®). The study had enrolled participants who had not previously received MS disease-modifying therapies (DMTs) and participants had monthly laboratory tests along with comprehensive testing every three months.

The study coordinator of the trial advised me that she was searching for someone to assist; I successfully applied for this position, which was being offered via the MS Society of Tasmania. And this was the beginning of my career as a MS specialist nurse.

When I was working in the infusion suite, I got to know a lot of the MS patients quite well because I loved chatting to them. These conversations and new acquaintances spurred me on to do a bit of extra research about MS and certainly generated a lot of interest for me to continue in the field. My previous experience within infectious diseases also demonstrated the unique perspective that a specialty nurse could bring to the area.

So for someone who had dodged a stock-broking job that could have landed them in Singapore, I came to find myself fast developing a dedicated career in multiple sclerosis. The CARE-MS trial led to a permanent position as one of the MS Specialist Nurses at the Royal Hobart Hospital's MS Clinic. Besides running the clinic, I was also working on three clinical trials in MS, including the ocrelizumab trial – a treatment for primary progressive MS – and also the PrevANZ study as well. The vitamin D MS Prevention Trial – or PrevANZ for short – is a world-first clinical trial that tests whether vitamin D supplementation can prevent or delay MS in those at risk of developing the disease.

In 2017, MS Research Australia funded the Australian MS Longitudinal Study (AMSLS) and the ensuing Economical Impact Report found that the prevalence of MS was the highest in Tasmania at 138.7 per 100,000 people, almost double that of other states such as Queensland at 74.6 per 100,000 and Western Australia at 87.7 per 100,000. The overall Australian prevalence of MS in 2017 was 103.7 people with MS per 100,000 people. So, despite being the smallest state or territory in Australia, we have the largest percentage of our population living with MS compared to other states in the country.

We had a great little team at the MS clinic and at MS Tasmania, and the neurologists would rely on us to be the gate keepers for people accessing the clinic and utilising the resources. And there was a lot of mutual respect amongst our team. As nurses we highly respected the decisions of the neurologists but similarly, the neuro's respected the advice and insights we could provide about the patients.

**

If someone had presented to the hospital whilst having an exacerbation and gone on to become diagnosed with MS, then I may have been one of the first health professionals to talk to these patients about MS and I would start educating them.

The newly diagnosed would most commonly ask if they could – or even should – have children? There was always that fear that everything in life was about to stop. They weren't necessarily thinking that MS would prevent them from having children, but more worried if they should have children for fear of passing the MS on. They also considered it selfish to have a child they may not be able to look after properly, especially if the MS progressed.

Most people would just fear that life in general would change overnight. Without a doubt, everyone had seen the advertisements of people with MS in wheelchairs and were just overwhelmed with the thought that they might have to immediately give up working or would become impaired in a flash.

It never helped that we couldn't separate the people in the MS clinic who were wheelchair bound. Hobart has a significant MS population, but the patients registered under our care obviously cover a multitude of disease stages. The shock factor was always there for a young 20-year-old – who might only be newly diagnosed or not even formally diagnosed – and you could see that they would be completely startled by wondering if this was their future? I have to admit there were times I'd just console the newly diagnosed by explaining we were running a gerontology study rather than confirming those people did in fact have MS. It was never easy trying to convince the newly diagnosed that their fate was not necessarily sealed just because of the variety of people they'd see in the clinic waiting room. But I can't deny how confronting it would be for people with MS – or any disease for that matter – to walk into a general MS clinic and wonder about their future. It's so terribly difficult not to compare yourself to others in that situation.

And I so often hear of patients who become freaked out by using specialists MS resources – such as physiotherapy or occupational therapy – because it can be too confronting to see people with progressive disability around them. Those patients who are living well with MS may also feel like they don't deserve to take up the resources from people who need them far more. But I actually find this a bit frustrating and try to convince my patients that if they in fact use the resources wisely now, then there's a very good chance they won't experience the type of severe progression they're seeing in the older patient cohorts. The uptake of resources that scare them are actually designed so as they can live the best life possible and will also save the health system a lot of money down the track because the patients have taken preventative measures now.

I spend a lot of time convincing my patients that 'their' job is to look after themselves now to the best of their ability and this responsibility involves a good diet, plenty of exercise and no smoking what-so-ever. I don't hold back any longer in reinforcing how it's not only the job of the person with MS to look after themselves, but in fact a priority.

The treatments we have for relapsing remitting MS are very good, but you still have to be living as a healthy human to reap the benefits; and especially for those people with MS who are in a progressive phase, it's essential they prioritise their health in the absence of choice of treatments. Let's face it, no amount of MS medication is going to reverse the effects or damage from smoking or obesity or a lack of general health and fitness.

***

People with MS understand we may not be able to fix everything – or even much at all – but they feel a sense of comfort and satisfaction when they've been heard.

Sometimes I do get very sad by what I see, particularly if I see a patient progressing with such a tremendous burden of disability. And for the most part, these patients really do just live for the moment. They are such an inspiration; to carry yourself that way when you could so easily crumble.

And there are so many people living with primary progressive MS that have become quite ingenious. They don't want anything to hold them back. I know one guy who loves his golf and he's had his golf clubs adjusted so he can hold them with an alternate grip. In fact, he's not long played on the Nullarbor Links, which has been dubbed the world's longest golf course. It's an 18-hole, par 72 golf course, spanning 1,365 kilometres, with one hole in each participating town or roadhouse along the Eyre Highway from Kalgoorlie in Western Australia to Ceduna in South Australia. For him, it was a lifelong dream.

It's hard to explain how I can find these people so inspirational and yet the situation can also make me sad. They don't let anything get in the way. Maybe I find it hard to reconcile in my mind that these people are doing amazing things for themselves (and often others) while carrying such a burden of disability and I can't help but wonder if they would be doing even greater things without that burden. But then I also have to wonder if they would have found that new respect for living life if they hadn't had been given the life-changing diagnosis of MS.

I'm often telling people to get on and live their life WITH MS, do not live a life OF MS. Yes... MS will be part of your life but please don't let it become all of your life.

But largely, I feel such joy when I see people who just work through the obstacles and get on with life.

Working as a MS specialist nurse has allowed me to become much more involved in the life of people living with MS. You become a person of support for them, and they look to you to help make sense of the disease with which they live. Unlike nursing on the wards at a hospital, where you nurse someone for a short period of time and they are discharged, the people I work with through the MS Society make regular contact with me, either through the MS clinic or via a phone consultation. The relationships you develop when you're a specialist MS nurse in this sort of environment tend to become ongoing, long term ones.

But ironically, one of the greatest reasons for loving my job also makes it one of the things I struggle with.

The 'good' is that I feel like I really get to know these people, and that's so enriching for me. But the 'bad' is that if something sad happens, I tend to feel the pain so deeply. And then there's sort of a mild mix of amusement and frustration in between all of that as well! Patients have telephoned me with the most insane requests at times, and when I query them as to why they'd be calling me – of all people – to help them with whatever they're calling about, they'll respond it's because they trust me. They tell me it's because I'm the person who actually listens to them and 'gets' them.

And that's a major thing I've noticed over the years. People with MS often just want to be listened to. They understand we may not be able to fix everything – or even much at all – but they feel a sense of comfort and satisfaction when they've been heard.

This need for connection and interaction may be an area where technology lets us down at times. A telephone helpline is a great solution for someone who just needs a quick answer. And people living in rural and remote areas do not always have access to specialist MS services, so the ability to speak with someone over the phone to have queries about symptoms and medications answered is essential. However, I know with my own patients, we have built up such a long and enduring relationship over time and explaining everything about their MS to a virtual stranger on the end of a telephone line can sometimes leave them a little frustrated: They want to speak with Michael! They know that I understand the quirks of their MS, and they take comfort in being able to discuss changes and potential solutions with me.

And for all the talking and listening that we do, and for the great variety of things that our patients and their families lean on us for, I do often feel the burden when we find ourselves in a position of acting as the psychologist. I'll personally stop my patients from treading that line and gently guide them that I can't help them with psychological queries; I ensure they understand I'm simply not the best person to help them in this field and that it's a bit beyond the boundary of my role. I am just not equipped with the skills to help people think in a different way, but I can help them find the mental health professional who is.

***

Understand the disease, because there's no doubt about it,
it's a fiendishly complex disease.

I think one of the key attributes of becoming a good MS nurse is quite basically, understanding the disease, because there's no doubt about it, it's a fiendishly complex disease. If you're going to become a specialty nurse in any disease, you have to get in there, and understand everything about it back-to-front. And I think along with that understanding also comes the ability to admit when you don't know, or don't have the answers, but are passionate enough to go off and find them.

And two of the most critical things in MS nursing are symptom knowledge and symptom management. The symptom management is something I've come to know inside out but every so often a weird little anomaly will pull me up. And some of that may also be because the internet plays such a large role in everyone's life now. In fact, Dr Google has become the bane of the MS nurse's life. Trying to help people make sense of the chat groups and some of the discussions that go on can be a very tricky thing. And I've had patients who get quite protective of their internet forums. They feel like it's 'their place' that they can talk to like-minded people and frankly, it's difficult to argue against their right to do so. The best we can do as nurses in this situation is direct them towards the reputable sites.

There's just so much 'white noise' out there now and we have a generation of patients coming through who are tremendously internet savvy. And I guess that's an enormous responsibility within our roles; to guide our patients in becoming educated about their disease and their health so as they can make informed decisions. I'd simply like to ensure my patients understand as much as they can and have as much information as possible so as they can make decisions about their own health and care. And sometimes they don't make the choices I wish they'd make, and no doubt also go against the advice of their neurologists, but so long as I feel they have understood the decision they are making then all I can do is reinforce that I'm still going to be there to stand beside them for assistance. And I have to be honest, when I first started doing this twenty years ago, I would never have thought that unravelling the white noise of a patient's resources would be part of my job.

I don't know that I can always reconcile some of the hard and heartbreaking things I see. And it does build up on you from time to time. I use a bit of black humour to deal with things. Maybe saying something a little dark and crazy is a release in itself? You've just got to try and find some way to lighten the situation. But we are surrounded by so much sadness and we have so much insight into how hard this disease can get, but for every one of those cases, I can share an example of the people who are living so positively and inspirationally and just outright full lives with the disease.

I bet that lady who took my arm at the volunteer's open day back in Melbourne over twenty five years ago could never have foreseen the career and life I've gone on to build... and passionately so. Isn't it funny how things turn out...

My hopes for the future treatment and management of MS:

• I feel the people being diagnosed with MS today have a great hope and opportunity of living a better quality of life, given the advances we've seen in treatment and symptom management.

• I've seen some great advancements – and with that great hope – in the treatment of MS during my career. Without a doubt, the introduction of the monoclonal antibodies as a treatment for people living with MS would be one of the most significant.

• In addition to the monoclonal antibodies, the introduction of oral treatments was also important. It may seem like such a small advancement, but the rates of compliancy amongst those needle-phobic patients was greatly lifted.

• And it's not just the treatment advancements but also the change in philosophy that have given people with MS the encouragement to live well. And as healthcare professionals, we feel a greater urgency to get a confirmed diagnosis and then discuss treatment options, because we know that people who are able to get onto a treatment earlier, experience better long-term results. And it feels so much better to be proactive, rather than sending our patients off with a promise to touch base in twelve months' time and see how they're feeling.

My advice for nurses beginning their career:

• Get to understand the disease the best you can because there's so many hidden symptoms that just can't be measured.

• Try and become as empathetic as you possibly can and understand what the patient is experiencing. I know we can only guess what living with MS and its various symptoms is like, but the more we know and the more we read and the more we talk to people, the greater our understanding will be.

• And most importantly, the more informed and empathetic you are, the greater your patients will trust you.

• There will be so many things you simply can't fix, but you can be there to listen to your patients and their carers and this is often one of the greatest salves.

• And finally, make sure you join your professional association. I have been a member of MS Nurses Australasia Inc for 10 years, and have met some of the most caring, knowledgable and hard woring nurses anywhere in Australia and New Zealand. I have made many good friends with members of this group, and they are only too happy to share their wisdom and ideas around MS nursing.

DEL THOMAS
Herefordshire, United Kingdom

"I like to say, 'a problem shared is a problem halved.'
It's what helps me go to sleep at night."

....

Well of course I was always going to go into nursing because I grew up hearing how fabulously glamorous it was! I was raised in the United Kingdom by Welsh parents and my mother's sisters were nurses and had achieved amazing careers. Both had emigrated to New York before I was born; one managed a private wing in a New York City hospital and nursed people like Gloria Vanderbilt and many other notorieties. I loved hearing all her stories. It was a great source of interest for me and I could only imagine how glamorous it must be. My aunt would also give me samples of the perfume that she'd been gifted by the people she nursed and regale me with the tales of the rich and famous. Of course, it wasn't until many, many years later that the reality of what nursing was actually like hit me! But by the time reality did hit, I was well and truly committed to becoming a nurse and in fact was very much encouraged by my family to pursue this career choice.

I started my nursing studies in 1987 and when I qualified, the British National Health Service (NHS) was a bit limited in that it only offered a fairly generic interview for placement in either a surgical ward or a medical ward. By default, I ended up in the medical ward. Back then, there really wasn't the formalised opportunity to choose a specialty. However, not long after I began my placement, I heard about a pilgrimage to Lourdes that had been organised and the trip was made up of MS patients; I was asked by one of my supervisors to assist. I have to say, it was phenomenal! We travelled on an adapted coach – and this was back in the '90s – and it had everything to make the trip incredibly comfortable and accessible for those with MS. We stayed at a fully-adaptive property near the pilgrimage site and had an amazing time.

On my return from this pilgrimage, I discovered I'd been transferred over to the medical respite and rehabilitation unit within neurology. Approximately eighty percent of our case workload in that unit was with people who were living with MS. The nature of the role meant that I was dealing with patients who clearly needed quite a bit of help and working in the respite unit launched me very quickly into understanding chronic illness and disability.

I developed a dedication and passion for learning about rehabilitation and respite and I became a sister in the unit within 18 months. And it was similarly that dedication that saw me stay in my role at Gloucestershire Royal Hospital for a decade.

But after ten years in rehab and respite, an opportunity arose to set up a new MS Relapse clinic. The NHS was starting the develop proper MS services because it was the dawn of a new era of treatments with the advent of the betaferon medications to treat MS. We'd never seen anything like the disease modifying therapies (DMTs) before and they needed to be stringently monitored. At the same time, we started seeing a lot more people dealing with multiple sclerosis who were younger and more able, and they certainly wanted to get on with life. These were the sort of patients who were keen to try the new betaferons and we had to embrace that within our services.

So I spent a year and a half researching these patient cohorts whilst also helping establish a new MS Relapse service at the Gloucestershire Royal Hospital. I published an article titled 'Improving service delivery for relapse management in multiple sclerosis' off the back of this research and shortly after I was also accredited as a MS specialist nurse.

After about three years of working in this acute environment as a MS nurse, an opportunity became available to develop a new MS service in the neighbouring county. However this time I was situated in a very rural setting. There was no big hospital with acute MS services; no neurologists who specialised in multiple sclerosis – only those with general neurology experience. The clinic would also be servicing a very different demographic given that most of the patients lived remotely in rural environments. But I decided from the beginning that I really wanted to embrace the challenge and start afresh. Although it wasn't really starting from scratch because I'd learned so much from setting up the previous clinic and was keen to put the new knowledge to work.

So in 2005 I found myself moving to Herefordshire, a small county in the mid-west of Britain and bordering on Wales. Tucked into the West Midlands, Herefordshire is one of the most rural and sparsely populated counties in England. With a population of approximately 191,000 – and the fourth-smallest of any ceremonial county in England – the area is well known for its fruit and cider production, and of course the Hereford cattle breed.

And fifteen years later I'm still here! Although admittedly it's been a challenge because of the nature of the county and the geography. Access to patients and providers can be difficult and I've had to be quite creative in how I dealt with that. One trick I discovered when I first started in the role, was to look at my patient's postal addresses and just from the postcodes I could identify the clusters of workloads

I needed to schedule.

When I first set the clinic up, the original patient load was quite low. Only some 150 patients in fact. But within a short time, I'd expanded to have around 600 patients. Clearly there were a lot more patients that were not being looked after and weren't accounted for within the specialised health services. Whilst newly diagnosed patients would provide a rationale for some of the increase, the quadrupling of people with MS can surely only be explained by the fact that patient numbers were originally under-recorded by the MS services and also being managed by local general practitioners but not reported to the National MS Society as having MS.

I quickly realised that a lot of education needed to be done in this county; not just for people living with MS but also for the benefit of the GPs and the hospitals. We needed to map out how to approach MS, how to treat relapses, how the disease could be managed. At that point in time, the GPs didn't even know how to go about obtaining an official diagnosis of MS. They were uncertain whether to refer straight onto a neurologist or obtain an MRI alongside that referral, let alone know how and when to refer a patient for greater disease management and provision of specialised services.

Initially I spent a lot of time educating our GPs and it's still something I continue today. I do worry that because I've been the specialist MS nurse in the county for over a decade that it's nearly a reflex action for providers to say 'just ring Del' in the situations where a patient presents with MS symptoms. I've seriously had situations where someone could be getting a breast screen and casually mention a MS-related concern to their GP, who will immediately refer them to me rather than assisting their patient with the easily-fixed complaint. If I can educate on what can be fixed in a GP's clinic by a family practitioner and what needs to be referred to a specialist, I think it would be far more efficient for everyone, and certainly much more advantageous for the person living with MS.

In those early days of setting up in Hereford County I sort of built a rod for my back because I encouraged the GPs to just ring me or refer directly to me for everything, but as the patient load grew I realised I just couldn't keep up with the work load and the burden grew. My patient time was being eaten away by returning calls and writing letters and it wasn't fair on anyone. Truthfully, I was sort of my own worst enemy! If I was to sustain the service and provide the best level of service to my patients then I needed to work out a way for the local GPs to take part-ownership of the MS patient care.

So the first thing I initiated was ensuring that every time I saw a patient, their local GP would get a written letter about the consultation, detailing what was discussed and the treatment or care plan we had established. The patient would also receive a copy so as everyone was literally on the same page. This also provided the patient a fair measure of comfort to know that their various health care providers were actively working on things and the clarity we created for all the stakeholders through this process was also a tremendous benefit. Basically, everything from this point on became a shared decision.

Years ago, if you had something wrong with you, you'd go to a doctor and be told what to do. But with MS, the situation is clearly very different. You can't tell people to just change their life; you can't tell people to just take this supplement or treatment and be on your way; you can't just say 'go exercise and that should help.' I think our job as MS nurses is to assist in manifesting these changes for the benefit of the person living with MS – and indeed their families – and by sharing the decisions and workload amongst all the care providers we can do this.

By establishing what the patient finds clear and also what their understanding is of their health and what their own priorities are in life, we build that rapport but importantly, we build a plan that suits them. Would it be easier to just tell the patient a laundry list of all the things they should do? Yes. Absolutely. But would it be optimal? No.

I find that some people do want to be given that list – or that firmer guidance if you will – but by and large we invest a lot of time in our consultations so we can really instil these longer lasting lifestyle changes in patients. In my consultations I'll often engage in techniques such as change talk and also utilise a lot of motivational interviewing styles to try and get people to understand the importance of making the changes necessary to their own conditions. We get them to visualise what these healthy changes would look like and how they would manage it. We get them to visualise how well-managed symptoms would manifest as a better and fuller lifestyle.

You're just not equipped with any of this knowledge when you first start the job of a MS nurse in the NHS. Primarily because there's not a lot of funding for education – of either the nurses or the patients – so in the UK we're very reliant on the MS Society, MS Trust and pharmaceutical companies to provide the MS professionals the additional education needed.

When it comes to multiple sclerosis in the United Kingdom, we probably have a multi-tiered health management and advocacy system much like other countries. We have the National Health Service (NHS), which is the publicly funded national healthcare system for England and one of the four national health services for each constituent country of the United Kingdom. It is the largest single-payer healthcare system in the world. Primarily funded through the general taxation collected by the government and overseen by the Department of Health and Social Care, NHS England provides healthcare to all legal English residents, with most services free at the point of use.

To fill in the support, care and educational gaps that the NHS doesn't provide are organisations such as the MS Trust and the MS Society. The Multiple Sclerosis Trust is an independent, national UK charity that was established in 1993. The MS Trust works to provide information for anyone affected by multiple sclerosis, education programmes for health professionals, funding for practical research, and campaigns for specialist MS services. A great deal of funding for MS specialist nurses comes from the MS Trust.

In fact, when a nurse commences work in multiple sclerosis services in the UK, they attend a one-week residential course within the first year in their position. The MS Trust have undertaken the facilitation of this to ensure a consistent level of expertise and training. It enables a wonderful networking experience and is enriching for the new nurses to share information and see how people work in the many and varied environments. And that's wonderful because no one person does it right. Everyone gets the information and interprets it slightly differently and then applies it to their clinics and patients. And that's wonderful for developing those adaptive skills. It's a phenomenal course.

Similarly, the MS Society is the UK's largest charity for people affected by MS. The member organisation funds research and provides education and training on MS to health professionals and those affected directly, as well as support to its 32,000 members via support groups and resources.

And I guess because of the under-resourcing from the NHS, we've had to go ahead and build what we need via other means. The United Kingdom MS Specialists Nurses Association (UKMSSNA) has been a great network of professional MS nurses empowering each other and sharing expertise. We've developed care manuals about symptoms and treatments and so many other online resources that are relevant in providing a high level of care in multiple sclerosis. And international collaboration has been key in developing these tools.

MS Nurses around the world all recognise that we work in different health care environments; our national health care systems could vary between countries, certainly the resources vary and most definitely the funding varies. But at the end of the day we're all treating people with MS. And as variable as the disease is amongst individuals, the commonality in how we provide clinical nursing support is the one thing that unites us. And in that sense, being able to bring some collaboration between colleagues nationally – and indeed internationally – is one of our most valuable resources and one of the accomplishments I'm most proud of.

***

MS doesn't inoculate you against everything else in life...

The type of questions my newly diagnosed patients will ask varies across the board. I get patients who come in and simply want to bury their head in the sand. It's important to note that in the UK we rarely see patients right at that point of diagnosis. Generally, what will happen is that a patient will be diagnosed at a hospital by a neurologist and then referred on to a MS nurse and a clinic at a later date, and the gold standard for this would be within four weeks from their diagnosis.

In the UK it is rare to have the MS nurses sit next to the neurologist or consulting specialist in the MS clinics to manage patients – and particularly the newly diagnosed – as a team. In my county we have two general neurologists who will diagnose my patients and then discharge them to me. Once I have the opportunity to consult to them and if I feel it necessary, I'll then refer them onto a neurologist who's a specialist in multiple sclerosis and we start building that support team of MS health professionals that way, which I understand is the opposite of other countries.

The National Institute of Health and Care Excellence (NICE) mandate that a Specialist MS nurse should see a person newly diagnosed with MS within four to six weeks of diagnosis. But that's still up to two months (or unfortunately longer in some cases) that a person has to refer to Dr Google or speak with other people (or people who know people) who have MS. And as nurses we realise there's comfort in speaking to others with MS and certainly empowerment in researching the disease yourself, but it needs to be done by the patient with an understanding that MS can be quite variable and individual amongst cases.

And don't forget that in some cases people recover quite well from those active symptoms and that initial flare; or on the other end of the spectrum it has taken a couple of years to become diagnosed after enduring many painful and unexplained symptoms.

So by the time we get to see them we're having to undo months – or even years – of misinformation, anger and confusion. The first thing I do when I have a new patient in front of me is to break down what has gone on to date so as I can formulate in my mind an approach that is going to be correct and tailored exactly for them. At that point I can explain why certain procedures have happened, why the diagnosis has taken a while or conversely why it's been quite fast. If I work my way through the diagnostic criteria, then I'll nearly always see the lightbulb moment as the person in front of me finally understands the process that has unfolded. This is that turning point where we'll start to unravel those misunderstandings of why someone else they knew had to have a lumbar puncture but they didn't or why they're on one type of medication but someone else is accessing another.

From then on, we can get into the type of questions that most people want to know; those factors that impact their lifestyle, such as the possibility of having children or hereditary concerns or workplace challenges right through to what the patient can do for themselves to manage the disease course.

Remember that by this time, most people – and their families – are feeling reasonably fed up with the diagnostic process. They've been in and out of hospitals for investigations and constantly visiting GPs and specialists to sort all these symptoms out. At this point they want to minimise any further hospital and clinical time and start sorting things out for themselves.

While two months may seem like an unreasonable time to wait to see your MS nurse, it's worth considering another theory. When you're first diagnosed with MS, do you actually absorb all the information at that point? I can visibly see when patients are just completely overwhelmed with too much information. But as a nurse we often have a set agenda in our head that we need to work through. And this doesn't always match what the person in front of us needs to hear at that point in time. But still we carry on talking for fear that we're not doing our jobs effectively, so we think we need to talk and talk and talk. But we don't. Often it's as simple as giving them a phone number and telling them what to do if things go belly up in those early days.

I think someone newly diagnosed with MS needs a bit of time to process what's going on. I don't necessarily believe that too much damage is done if we're not seeing the patient within ten minutes of diagnosis. But really, there's no right or wrong…. It's just something I like to philosophise about.

As specialist nurses we'll have a checklist in our head of items to run through and then the patient will have their own checklist of things they want to discuss and very rarely do those two lists marry up! There's quite a skill in working out how to unite those disparate lists at the start of any consultation. It takes time to develop that skill and also having confidence in yourself.

Knowing how much information to impart and when, becomes intuitive over time. And knowing who to give the information to is also part of that equation.

I always coach my patients that in the first year they are going to analyse every little thing that goes on in their body. So I'll implore them to think of everything else first and their MS last because having MS doesn't inoculate you against everything else in life. For the newly diagnosed, if they have something wrong, they're automatically going to assume it's the MS. The newly diagnosed need to learn that everything in the first year is going to be a learning curve; they weren't created with an inbuilt MS manual and they'll need to learn as they go along, and particularly learn how to pace themselves. They learn through life and each person will actually end up writing their own individually tailored manual on how they manage the disease.

***

An evolution in how people cope with MS

It's great to have support but there's good support and bad support. And then there's support groups to add into the mix. And so many aspects of living with MS have changed quite dramatically over the years and I'm really conscious of trying to have people find their own support network. Some of the organised support groups may be great for people with a certain type of lifestyle or at a certain stage of disease course, but that same group may not be the most ideal place for a newly diagnosed person.

And on the topic of MS changing, we're teaching the younger and newly diagnosed patients to manage better earlier; to get ahead of the disease if you will. Ten years ago, I may have had a lot of contact with patients and now, I find a great deal of people with MS are just living with it so well that they don't need the full-on support we once had to provide. It's been nothing short of an evolution of how people cope with MS.

The newer support models found in the online blogging and social media platforms mean that the face-to-face groups are becoming antiquated for those younger patients. And whilst the established support groups will always serve a purpose for those longer-term members – perhaps providing benefits more of a social nature – those types of traditional groups simply don't have the skills to guide the newly diagnosed any longer.

And I ponder how advocacy and charity groups around the world – not just in the United Kingdom – will really start to experience some fundamental issues in how they maintain and sustain a relevancy with their key stakeholders when the disease has changed so much over the last decade alone due to better diagnostic techniques and treatments.

Multiple sclerosis is also becoming quite politicised in the UK. Here we have an all-party parliamentary group of which the MS Society are the secretariat, so often the parliamentary agenda around multiple sclerosis is pre-designed by the MS Society. However, the Society doesn't always engage with the health professionals to present a fully balanced and contemporary view of MS in this country. I've been to parliament on five occasions and I've spoken about the role of MS nurses in the UK and the importance of our role in managing MS and the drug treatments. And I've found that while the Society does a great job in many areas, the information presented to parliament to further our cause doesn't quite hit the mark. This is a by-product of not engaging with the people most appropriately positioned to provide the frontline advice or the fact that they may not have asked the right questions to compile reporting information.

I'll give you a recent example: In the UK we have a process called postcode prescribing. So one area of the country will have fantastic services whilst another part of the country won't have such great service. One of the questions on a survey that the Society undertook was to self-report the type of MS the respondent had. That's fine but if you haven't seen a neurologist in 15 years then you may not have much of an idea. It was a very poorly worded questionnaire and I believe that the results would have delivered a report that was not entirely true and accurate.

We have loads of wonderful literature in the UK and in general the support we can provide the patients is due largely to the work of the MS Trust, the UK MS Society and the NHS. And I can honestly say that I couldn't do my work as a MS Nurse today without the work of the MS Trust. I also know from the anecdotes of my colleagues that these systemic problems are faced the world around; regardless I find them frustrating at times.

***

There's Never Enough Time: Frustrations and Challenges

Resources, money and time. Show me an MS nurse anywhere in the world who doesn't experience frustration because of the lack of any of those. For me in the UK, I find that the NHS in itself is systemically restricting because we haven't generally been able to engage them in wanting to expand community MS services. The big specialist centres tend to be very invested and focussed on providing the infusion DMTs and by the very nature of that, those centres are often getting significant funding injections from the pharmaceutical companies as well. And by the very volume of patients that these larger city centres see, there's just more money put into the clinics. It's not rocket science or illogical. But in our rural clinics, we don't get the same opportunities or nature of funding to be able to expand. And to me that's a travesty because the type of care we need to provide in our MS centres regionally is as acute and imperative as in the city centres; I daresay more so. And we tend to be with the patient over the lifetime of the disease, rather than just treatment-to-treatment.

And this concerns me greatly, particularly in a day and age when so many people are moving back into regional areas. They move back to be near family, to escape the city, to live a more relaxed lifestyle or find that healthy sea change. It's been supremely frustrating that the NHS doesn't recognise that the community and MS teams within those rural settings are vitally important too and should be invested in.

Our psychological services for neurological patients are also minimally supported by the NHS. In the case where there's cognitive decline in a patient, their ability to make good decisions may be compromised. We come across some patients who ethically sit on that boundary of high risk, perhaps because of their mental health or cognitive disability.

I have patients who deal with a variety of health issues that may impact greatly on their MS from the point of view that they have mental health challenges or cognition difficulties and they can't process the approach we're trying to instil in them to manage the MS. Treating people who have those level of cognitive impairment challenges can be difficult, particularly if the support network isn't there to assist them and finding the best structures or programme to provide the support they need can be demanding. We don't want to see people with MS go into nursing homes and luckily, we're able to avoid that in a lot of cases. But with so many restrictions to the amount of services the NHS can provide, we don't always get the amount and level of care for those greatest in need.

But my other great frustration is simply time. We just don't have enough time in the day to do what we want. There's just not enough of us. In the whole of the UK I think there's around 240 MS specialist nurses for some 110,000 people living with MS. There's been a dawn of a new type of MS nurse over the last few years and that's been largely encouraging but also throws up some new challenges. With the introduction of the infusion centres, we now have nurses who qualify as infusion nurses and then of course in the MS centres we have clinical nurse specialists. And the infusion nurses will have their own challenges in managing infusion schedules and patient treatment protocols for the various DMTs. And it's not just about the treatment procedure because they've still got the person in front of them who is living with MS; and obviously to most people with MS, a nurse is a nurse and they will offload on the nurse standing in front of them about a range of concerns. And these infusion nurses may not necessarily have the skills or the time to effectively help the MS patient. And a loftier question to ask is if it's even the role of the infusion nurse to deal with these concerns?

The Wye Valley MS Clinic system cares for approximately 600 patients in the area. We manage our primary clinic in Hereford and then also go out into the regional community hospitals for additional clinic days. Overall I average four to five clinics a week. Then I'll also undertake telephone consultations and manage a telephone help line, consult in the care and management of the newly diagnosed, do home visits and monitoring of all the drugs we administer. Up until very recently I had to do most of this by myself but we've just added another MS nurse to the clinic and that's been wonderful.

Across the board and as a general observation, I'm also very conscious that the patients who are taking a MS treatment – and particularly those taking the newer DMTs – are getting regular and constant monitoring. However, for those patients who are not on any drugs, either because they're in a progressive disease stage or can't take the drugs for one reason or another, they basically get reduced contact, specifically from the bigger centres, due to their capacity constraints. I'm personally of the opinion that I need to see everybody with MS in my county, no matter whether they have relapsing remitting, primary progressive or secondary progressive forms of MS. Within the service I oversee, I'm extremely careful that I don't allow these patients to fall between the cracks. Somehow, I'm determined to keep my other patients – those who are ineligible for the DMTs – feeling engaged and committed to our appointments together, so we can aim for better symptom management and to discuss new research and lifestyle choices and just to let them know they're not alone in this.

But patients on the DMTs simply need more frequent clinic appointments. In the case of a DMT such as Lemtrada, I need to see a patient every month for four years after their second infusion. So this could be up to six years of monthly appointments for a single patient. And if I have up to twenty patients on that DMT alone, that's two to three clinic days a month fully scheduled to monitor patients on just one type of drug available. It's becoming very easy for the MS nurses to be (wrongly) perceived as being purely a drug servicing nurse in the UK, particularly given the lack of investment by the NHS to grow the MS services as a whole to support every patient with MS adequately.

It's really hard to attend to the small details when you're managing the big picture in all of this. I think I fail at managing all the telephone consultations I want to do. I can deal with the face-to-face appointments and the home visits and luckily, I have administrative support to assist with the many scripts for the DMTs and associated blood monitoring and to also type up the dictated letters I send back to the various health professionals. I'm very fortunate to have this admin help because there's many, many nurses around the UK who don't have that support and desperately need it. And the minutia of admin is such a waste of the time and expertise of the MS nurse and takes away from the patient contact time. And there's certainly an economic impact to that.

Let's put it into perspective. If I see on average forty patients per week, that's forty letters that need to be composed and then typed. Even at a conservative twenty minutes per letter, that's over thirteen hours a week of admin work. It's ridiculous!

When you're managing the volume of patients that we are, it can be difficult to work out where the priorities need to lie; to work out which patient needs your attention over another. And ideally you wouldn't even have to be making these choices but it's an unfortunate and common reality. And like anything in life, those who shout the loudest often get that attention. But for me, it's imperative that every patient – no matter their disease stage – are seen once a year as a minimum.

***

A problem shared is a problem halved...

To be honest, I could worry about a great many of my patients. They're not just a medical chart to me. I go into their homes and see how they live; I know about their family dynamics, and I have good handle on their mental health. Over the course of my 24 years in MS nursing I've seen and heard just about everything. From those patients who get themselves in terrible binds with the disease to those who just want to give up and go to Switzerland where it's legal to seek assisted suicide.

But I learned years ago not to go home and go to bed and keep myself up all night worrying about things. Regardless, it's a huge burden on one person. So this sharing of information – whether it be amongst my peers or between the patient's team of health professionals – is my way of ensuring the burden is shared. I like to say, 'a problem shared is a problem halved.' It's what helps me go to sleep at night.

MS nurses in the UK work hard and we also network extremely well, which is tremendously beneficial for us in both a professional and social sense. Having that social outlet amongst peers is just so important. We can all go home to our family and partners and offload about the day, but our family can often only listen, and try as they might, they can't offer concrete advice because they won't understand the peculiarities of our jobs. But my colleagues unequivocally understand and generally without judgment! They understand the parameters and constraints you deal with at every turn and the nuances of treatment that these new DMTs bring to our roles.

With every new drug there's another new challenge to tackle and another challenge of finding the time to fit that in on top of everything else we've already got going on. And amongst our peers we don't need to verbalise these frustrations because we're all in the same boat. It's reassuring but also quite relaxing to be amongst peers because you know everyone is feeling the same type of burden and responsibility as you.

The burden of monitoring the DMTs is enormous. The new breed of DMTs are proving to be wonderful at dampening disease and halting progression but they can be nasty drugs that do pretty radical things. And the burden with making sure we get it right and 'do no harm' weighs heavily on me.

And that's when it becomes very important to be able to offload to your colleagues about this burden.

***

My career as a MS nurse has changed my life in so many more ways than I could imagine. It didn't turn out to be all Gloria Vanderbilts and wafting around the wards with glamorous bottles of perfume. Although I did do tea at the Queen's Garden Party not so long ago....

But it's been enriching from day one. It's given me a sense of confidence and empowerment I never dreamed I could cultivate from a profession like this. And it's taught me so many valuable (and amusing) lessons in life. And after more than 25 years of working in MS, the passion I have is so deeply rooted in my fibre that I couldn't imagine it any other way.

My hopes for the future treatment and management of MS:

•   The biggest advance I've seen throughout my career as a MS nurse is certainly the development and introduction of the DMTs. The introduction of the DMTs has meant that the MS services have had to expand and without the DMTs we may not have facilitated those expansion of services. However, the introduction of the DMTs has made our role so complex and there are so many different DMTs available now that our more traditional MS services have had to morph into drug administration and monitoring services, without capacity to see progressive patients. So on one hand, the biggest wonder has been the introduction of more robust drugs to treat MS but it's also been our biggest downfall. It's been a very tricky balance to strike and will continue to be so, well into the future. And I'm sure the UK won't be unique in facing these challenges.

•   I don't even think about the word 'cure' because I truly believe we need to identify more about the disease and gain a greater understanding of what actually causes multiple sclerosis.

•   And I don't talk about a cure at all when I'm talking to people with MS. I just don't want to give people false hope. And hope is talked about a lot because we all need hope in life. I'd rather talk about current research that is going on; I'd rather be very realistic and pragmatic with the people I see.

•   The other great advantage to understanding more about MS is that I believe we'll be able to strive towards matching our patients to the treatments. We're on the frontier of personalised medicine with more DMT's being developed to combat particular symptoms of MS but I think if we understood more about what causes MS, we could do so much better at marrying up people to treatments.

My advice for nurses beginning their career:

- One of the things I've learned over the years is not to discount a patient's own research and the work they invest into themselves. Even if I don't agree with some of the suggestions – say for example the suggestion that turmeric lattes help with their aches and pains – then I'm happy to go along with this as the patient is unlikely to do any harm to themselves.

- In these instances, I won't dismiss a patient's own suggestion too hastily. I won't laugh back that something isn't recognised by the NHS or that neurological studies prove x, y and z. My response would be more along the lines that I'm really happy they've taken some time to research and invest in their own health and that I'm sure that part of the process of researching how to manage their own health is mentally beneficial as well; that there's a benefit in taking a bit of control. So whilst some of these remedies may not be physically beneficial in managing symptoms and lacking in evidence, there's a benefit psychologically.

- I would also encourage implementing and maintaining a well-scheduled day. I'm very strict with the structure of my day and how I've adapted my service so as I have set clinics and a set time when I'll do home visits then I also diarise a set time each week when I'll look at blood monitoring, a set time to do my phone calls. I'm very structured in the approach to my time so that I can maximise what is achievable.

- And the other thing I'm always aiming to do is to go home on time. I may sound counter-intuitive given the burdensome case load we manage but going home on time is my way of looking after myself. I may come into the clinic at a ridiculous-o'clock in the morning, but I always aim to get home on time at night!

SUSAN AGLAND
Newcastle, Australia

When we lose specialist MS nurses, it's like losing the lifeforce of our MS community. The knock-on effect simply can't be under-estimated.

....

I'm a born and bred Novocastrian – the eldest of two children – and the seed was planted very early that I would eventually become a nurse. So early in fact, that when my mother was pregnant with me, her mother-in-law adamantly proclaimed this first-born child would be a girl, and the girl would go on to be a nurse. Mum's mother-in-law was a matron of nursing who forged her own career in the pre- and post-war era of the 1940s. She was nothing if not without military-like precision and timing, which is very clearly a different style to the type of nursing work I do now! But the foundation of her nursing practice back then was all about looking after the whole person, not just the fracture or the infection. This ideal of caring was demonstrative in the care of her granddaughters. I feel it's something I've grown up with; perhaps that's why providing holistic care is such a focus for me. The military-like approach had its down sides. We were discouraged from lying around (there was no such thing as lounging) and everybody was expected to contribute – everyone had a job to do.

So I actually started nursing as a toddler! I would attend to my grandfather – completely decked out in a little nurse's uniform – and ensuring his wounded leg or scratched arm was all bandaged up and taking his temperature to determine whether he would live or die. I just knew I never wanted to do anything else.

The most important thing I learnt from my parents and grandparents was that I could do anything. If I wanted to do something, all I had to do was have a go. They put their money and support behind me – paying for piano lessons and choir tours, driving me to rehearsals and going without so I could do. Skip ahead now and that mantra is central to my life and the life lessons I pass on to my children. You can do anything if you put your mind to it. Have a go and don't let the 'what if I can't' stop you. Say yes and worry about how you're going to do it later. Ultimately, that's why I said yes to MS when the opportunity presented itself.

My ingrained sense of holistic care also extends through to the community work I immerse myself into. But that's just how we were brought up as kids; no way could you sit around on your backside if there was a hand to be lent somewhere! So taking all these early learning experiences and inbuilt characteristics into a nursing practice was fairly natural to me; but to get paid for doing it as well was a complete bonus!

After my undergraduate degree at the University of Newcastle I continued nursing in my hometown. In my first year out, I was thrown into the deep end and straight into neurology; or more precisely neurosurgery and neuro-rehabilitation. I was also one of the first group of university-trained nurses to transition from the practical-based nursing training model to being university-trained and we were really put through our paces. Every day we'd have to prove our worth in how well we could make a bed and discern what was going on with our patients without relying on stats and figures.

And you know, that's fine.... it was all a rite of passage. Frankly, nurses have a habit of eating their young so there wouldn't be too many nurses out there who weren't hazed or put to the test in some way! I really believe you can take on the world if you survive your first year of nursing. And hey...I haven't left the specialist field of neurology since, so it couldn't have been too bad!

The first decade of my career was in neurosurgery and whilst it was phenomenally amazing, it was also exhausting. The field involves an incredible amount of shift work and years of pushing through double shifts was a formidable challenge both emotionally and physically.

And the nature of neurosurgery is that you're dealing with people who have been through some pretty horrendous situations and the resulting surgeries can be very hard and pronounced on their moods and personalities afterwards. All in all, we would deal with exceptionally acute cases, and it was always going to get to a point that was more than I could bear. After a decade – and despite knowing I was part of something really wonderful and working with a team of brilliant people – I just found it exhausting on my soul.

Around this time, the opportunity arose to do a temporary secondment with one of the neurologists as the Newcastle site nurse for the AusImmune study. I figured this deviation into 'research land' would be the perfect sojourn to alleviate the burn-out I was feeling. And I couldn't wait to catch up on a decade of missed sleep!

The Australian Multi-centre Study of Environment and Immune Function (the AusImmune Study) is a multi-centre, case-control study investigating the role of environmental factors in the development of first demyelinating events (FDEs), a frequent precursor to multiple sclerosis. The environmental factors include past and recent sun exposure (and vitamin D levels), viral infections, chemical exposures, diet, and genetic factors.

The AusImmune Study is the first observational epidemiological study to be able to provide population-based incidence data for early demyelinating disease across a broad latitudinal gradient (from more northern to southern parts of Australia) encompassing considerable environmental diversity, within a uniform health care system. As such, Australia provides a unique opportunity to do this work.

My work on AusImmune was really fascinating and would last for approximately eighteen months before I was asked to become the MS nurse in a new MS clinic that was to be opened at the John Hunter Hospital in Newcastle.

While the move across to the MS clinic was an obvious and welcome transition for me, I couldn't help but second guess if I was doing the right thing in leaving the highly-skilled field of neurosurgery and the brilliant colleagues who'd become firm friends in the time I'd spent there. But during my secondment at AusImmune, I found that I'd built up such a good rapport and interest in the MS patients I was seeing with Clinically Isolated Syndrome (CIS) and I thoroughly enjoyed the work.

And if I was being honest with myself, what I thought would be a bit of a 'vacation' job from neurosurgery to recharge the batteries was actually something that challenged me and resonated deeply. And not once, in those thirteen years since, have I wished I'd gone back to my old job.

***

*Patients who embrace self-management do so much better
from the onset. They have this look in their eyes that they
want to get on with life.*

The John Hunter Hospital MS Clinic opened in May 2006 and we
have grown year after year; it seems that prevalence and incidence of
MS is increasing everywhere. We are the largest MS centre in New
South Wales, and certainly one of the largest centres in Australia
with a little over 1,000 patients registered with us. We have clinics
every day of the week, at two campuses; John Hunter Hospital and
Belmont Hospital. We have a great, although small clinical team of
3 doctors, a very busy but caring admin and myself. We work closely
with a larger and very involved MS research team of PhD students,
post docs, clinical trial staff and a research nurse.

Our location two and a half hours north of Sydney means that we
are the only major centre between Sydney and the Gold Coast, so
we naturally attract clients from all those rural and regional locations
in between – such as the upper Hunter Valley, the north coast and
Tamworth and Armidale – but we also have a lot of patients and
families who come in from the west of the state because they find it
easier to travel to Newcastle rather than venture into Sydney. More
than one third of our patients have to journey greater than an hour to
visit us. In fact, we have patients who routinely drive four hours for
their care and there are some who make an eight-hour trip. At times,
I can't help but think we have such a backward system for providing
care to the huge number of patients who have no alternative but to
travel great distances as they have no services closer to their home.

My day-to-day role at the MS clinic is simply to keep people
well and out of hospital. That means counselling, educating and
getting people on to the right treatments for them: drug treatments
and non-drug treatments. Monitoring and managing the 'on-drug'
experience is important. The newer therapies are very effective

but that comes with an increased risk of side effects. I also triage new symptoms, to bring MSers into hospital if necessary but also to manage relapses in the outpatient setting. This setting might not be in my hospital network, but rather regional services, so developing and supporting these professional networks is vital to keeping people working, living and receiving care in their local area. In the last few years, helping people access the National Disability Insurance Scheme (NDIS) and Disability Support has become a significant wedge of my time. I like and loath the paperwork; sometimes it feels like the larger system just doesn't get MS but it's important MS nurses advocate. Sometimes we just need to be the pain in the backside of the agency we are trying to access support from, for our patients. I suspect most MS nurses are alike in this respect: when facing nonsensical rejection, a little piece of me enjoys being the pain in the agency's backside.

Basically, from the minute a person is diagnosed (or even going through the diagnostic process) I will be part that patient's life in the MS clinic. I meet them on the wards in those early days and re-assure them that I will be there – and be their main point of contact moving forward – for anything they may need. I want to be there to answer questions, work with them through treatments issues, help them with symptom management.... anything to try and pull the puzzle together for them.

But having said that, something I'm really passionate about is promoting a patient's self-management. I find the first year or two are the most crucial in helping the newly diagnosed come to terms with things, and they need support to sift and sort their way forward. They are encouraged to call or email as and when they need to. Then, they start to see above the fog and become a bit more confident that they can manage this disease and they can start to take control. I know when people have 'got it' because I start hear to less and less from them. It's something I encourage people to reflect on – the not needing to call for advice. Because it means they have adapted, they have it in hand. They know they can call anytime, a bit like a safety net.

Let's face it: Right up until the symptoms manifested or the person was 'officially' diagnosed with MS, they were already self-managing in life. And most of them pretty well!

But then along comes MS and we rip the carpet out from underneath them, telling them that they are now living with a chronic disease and that life will change and there's all this new information and scenarios and even life skills to take on board. And we deliver all of this with an unfortunate degree of uncertainty around what actually might or might not happen during their own disease course.

So quite simply, I don't want to take away someone's ability (or right) to try and self-manage their care; I just want to help them cultivate a new-found confidence and proficiency to live well, despite MS. And deep down, I also know that the patient with MS will always know their MS better than I will in the coming years! They're the one living with it, they have an innate sense of when something's not right, so to develop those new self-awareness and self-management muscles early gives them every opportunity to continue living life the way they want to. I mean, imagine feeling as if you need to check in with a doctor about every single little thing you want to do? Or feel as if you needed some type of permission to go somewhere different to the norm. Who wants that?'

Patients who embrace self-management do so much better from the onset. They have this look in their eyes that they want to get on with life.

***

"Are you sure?"

I was trying to think what it is the newly diagnosed ask the most in those first few uncertain months and the most frequent question is not necessarily about treatments or lifestyle or what-have-you, but simply "are you sure?" It pulls me up in my tracks every time. My patients may not necessarily have been shown the MRI's or lumbar puncture results or blood tests by their neurologist in those early days – and the patients won't know to ask for them – so there's no visual evidence to help the patient process or comprehend the news of the diagnosis. I'm often quizzed to make sure it's not something else altogether, such as a tumour or a virus. They'll explain they may not have been eating well and that life had become stressful so maybe it's a vitamin deficiency or something they did to themselves? They just want to make sure we've got it right.

I know it may be a hard thing to fathom, but I've heard too many times about how a patient will be admitted to a hospital's ER with symptoms indicative of MS – often on a Friday afternoon. They'll have an emergency MRI and then someone else on the ward will deliver the blunt results to the patient. "You have MS." As simple and blunt as that, then striding out, leaving the shocked patient alone all weekend, without family, friends or really any relevant support. It's horrendous!

Myself, and the neurologist I work with, Professor Jeannette Lechner-Scott, will take the time to sit down with our patients and work through all of these key pieces of information together; I really feel it's a crucial exercise and part of the very important education process.

The next big question after "are you sure?" is "well what do I do now?" And "how do I know what to do when?" My philosophy, which I explain to patients in those early days, is that they may need us a lot now, but we ultimately help them create the knowledge and tools to move forward. And I find patients are always hyper-vigilant at this stage for any new problems and there's understandably an awful lot of handholding in those first twelve months.

Dr Google plays enough havoc in the management of our patients that we have recently produced a brochure for people who become diagnosed on the wards, and particularly during the weekend, where there's no immediate MS nursing support. We wanted to guide these newly diagnosed and their family towards the reputable and frankly hopeful places where people could search for information, at least in the interim to our consultations.

It's human nature to want answers as soon as possible and we just want to try and quell the fear and provide some small pieces of reputable information in the heat of the moment. The other key message we're trying to convey in the brochure is – first and foremost – not to panic! This diagnosis is not life threatening or life ending; help will be at hand and we can guide you in this process. We have actually taken to imploring our new patients not to go looking for any other information until they have spoken with our specialist MS team.

That notion of time is a really big topic to contemplate. Everything probably feels like it's colliding or imploding for someone newly diagnosed with MS, but it can be so beneficial to understand that you have time; you have a moment to just think and recalibrate. Taking some time to consider options and clear the headspace is a rational way to proceed.

And the concept of time will mean different things to different people. We know that getting patients onto an appropriate MS treatment early is highly effective in preventing disease progression but starting a treatment will happen when they're ready. I often say to my patients that 'your concept of ready doesn't have to be someone else's concept of ready.'

***

The telehealth service we provide obviously reduces the amount of travel for people, which is very important in our mission to make it as easy as possible for our patients to maintain regular check-ups with the clinic. While there are still lots of appointments where the neurologist will need to lay hands on their patients for an objective assessment, we might suggest using the telehealth system every second appointment or so, especially if it reduces the burden on the patient or their family. And Australia's publicly funded universal health insurance scheme, Medicare, will often assist with the cost of the telehealth consultation for those people who live quite remotely.

Our standard routine is to see our patients every six months for a check-up, whether they're well and stable or not. Patients with greater health concerns are seen as frequently as they need to be, particularly those who might be relapsing more often and we're wanting to alleviate the concerns and anxiety they're feeling, as well as making sure they are on the right drug for their disease.

But telehealth is a great tool that can assist us monitoring the people who are living very well with MS. Living with and managing MS can be expensive and time consuming, so our clinic has embraced telehealth as a way to minimising some of those pressure points for people. At the very least they're not having to take a full day or two off work, sit in a car for hours on end and having to spend the night in another city.

It's a system that works really well for the families in regional areas and we've now found that some patients who live in close proximity to each other might co-ordinate and all travel to the clinic together, making a 'girl's trip' out of the face-to-face check-ups or treatments.

I think my greatest frustration as a MS nurse remains that we tend to work in a limited system with limited funding. Working in a public hospital system has its own challenges and I often question how much value they see in what we do. There are never enough consultation times to review every patient the way we want to. We need more time, more resources, more specialist nurses, and I find that within the public hospital system, it comes down to a limited bucket of money for a rapidly growing population with increased needs.

Every day I have to be extremely creative in my problem solving. A good example of this might be how I'm going to engage with a rural health care centre to deliver a service for a patient in their own region, so as the patient doesn't have to travel to Newcastle. Often we're asking these providers to administer a service they may never have done before; we might need to get some of these smaller ambulatory care centres to provide an infusion service. Sometimes we hit the jackpot and they will do whatever it takes (even with already stretched resources) and other times it's difficult for services to see beyond the limitations of their own systems. I find it supremely frustrating when I'm confronted with a 'it's not my job' or 'yeah, nah, we don't do that here' kind of attitude.

Maybe advocating for nurses at a higher level is one of the ways I subconsciously deal with these systemic frustrations? Unfortunately, in Australia we have continued to lose funding for specialised MS nurses and a few years ago when I was the president of the MS Nurses Australasia (MSNA), rectifying this problem was something I fought for passionately. But it was tough... MS is not seen as a high-priority disease to deal with in Australia; we don't have a high-profile media hook and it's not seen as a condition that effects a lot of people, despite the statistics telling us that one in four people in Australia know someone or have a loved one living with the potentially debilitating condition.

When we lose specialist MS nurses, it's like losing the lifeforce of our MS community. The knock-on effect simply can't be under-estimated. It's inconceivable to think we could replace a nurse who has forged ten or twenty-plus years' experience in supporting people with MS, with a generalist or an online solution. I actually worry very deeply about this issue.

***

I get more out of MS nursing than I give.

The patient is always at the forefront of my mind and anything I do is because I keep the interests of my patients front and centre. Sometimes this gets me in a spot of trouble! I don't set out to be contentious or confrontational, but I just think I have a great opportunity to make the lives of people living with MS quite manageable and full of hope.

I'm probably an excellent case study in how NOT to find balance. I do take it all home; it becomes all-consuming and I become completely engrossed in things at ridiculous hours. Unsurprisingly, other things in my life can suffer at times. I have to be honest; I feel like when I'm at work, I'm a terrible Mum and wife. And when I'm at home I'm a terrible MS nurse. So, no, balance isn't a concept I do well.

But I enjoy being really busy and anyone who knows me, knows I can't sit still! And if I can see something that needs changing, you better believe I'll be up for giving it a red hot go. I'm constantly tired and I'm checking emails at all hours of the night and on weekends, but I can assure in no uncertain terms, that I get more out of MS nursing than I give. It pays dividends to me personally that most wouldn't understand. I have forged, not just a job but a career out of MS nursing.

The amazing people I've met over the years have given me so much strength to push through the hard times. I have the friendship of my peers in Australia, NZ and around the world that I can turn to, but on the flipside of the coin, I draw so much inspiration from my patients who are doing it tough, but doing so with grace and courage.

My historical tendency of not being able to manage stress actually led me to pursue my research masters with a focus on whether stress management programmes can reduce stress and improve the quality of life in people diagnosed with multiple sclerosis. I'd come across the works of an American researcher, Professor David Mohr, who's written extensively about stress and mood management programmes for people with MS. He is particularly well-known for developing and evaluating technology-assisted behavioural and psychological interventions and researching the relationship between stress, depression and inflammation in multiple sclerosis patients.

Back in the early 2000s, he undertook a clinical trial which examined the efficacy of a stress management program in reducing neuroimaging markers of multiple sclerosis disease activity. A total of 121 patients with relapsing forms of MS were randomised to receive a manualised stress management therapy (SMT-MS) – essentially meditation and mindfulness for MS – or instead a wait-list control condition. SMT-MS provided 16 individual treatment sessions over 24 weeks, followed by a 24-week post-treatment follow-up. The primary outcome was the cumulative number of new gadolinium-enhancing (Gd+) brain lesions on MRI at weeks 8, 16, and 24. Secondary outcomes included new or enlarging T2 MRI lesions, brain volume change, clinical exacerbation, and stress.

This study provided Class I evidence that SMT-MS reduced the number of Gd+ lesions in patients with MS during the 24-week treatment period. Interestingly, the gains made after this initial period where often lost and Mohr concluded it was because trial participants had ceased the regular stress management techniques. Other studies at the time also showed that managing stress brought about reduced perceived stress levels, improved adjustment to having a chronic disease and improved quality of life.

It was truly an eye-opening discovery for me because I realised that teaching mindfulness and meditation was something that MS nurses could learn to do in existing nurse roles and clinics. The benefit to our patients would be well worth it. As nurses, our patients tend to confide in us and accept our guidance; we're in a great position to be able to introduce the stress management techniques and it involves tools that are freely available.

My study, 'Managing Stress in MS,' found trends for improved quality of life, but statistical significance was not achieved. The population of people it did work for was those who already had some exposure to the stress management strategies or who were open to the idea of mindfulness and regular meditation. Echoing what the other studies had shown, was that one strategy doesn't work for all and secondly, when you stop making managing stress a daily habit, people revert to old habits.

The masters research project has really shown me the personal benefit of practicing mindfulness every day. I'm a terrible meditator but the mindfulness is a great stabiliser in my life, particularly given everything I juggle. I keep promising myself that I will try to be a better meditator!

The other game-changing technique and something I love to speak with my patients about is reframing the challenges we face, something akin to the way cognitive behavioural therapy does. I think when you can put things into perspective, you'll inherently learn how to cope better with the change that MS and life in general throws at us. And our research in the master's project kept proving this to us time after time. We saw that if someone could learn to reframe MS from the outset, if they could work through things from the practical perspectives rather than becoming caught up in the emotional ones. Put simply, those people that attempted to reframe the challenges seemed to be able to get on with the things they could do (and enjoy them) and not worry so much about the things they couldn't change.

The international standardisation for what we should consider achievable benchmarks for the timing of key events in the MS care pathway – or MS Brain Health standards for short – are another area in my recent career that I believe are vitally important. It is simply the gold standard in how we can maximise lifelong brain health.

Brain health should be valued highly, as it helps people maintain a good quality of life as they age, and the MS Brain Health initiative highlights the need to maximise lifelong brain health by making recommendations to monitor and minimise disease activity.

According to the MS Brain Health initiative, the brain is a remarkably flexible organ. If MS disease activity damages tissue in one area, other areas can work harder to compensate. This extra capacity is known as 'neurological reserve', or 'brain health', and explains why disease activity may go undetected during the early phase of MS. Indeed, cognitive problems may develop before more obvious symptoms of MS appear – sometimes years earlier.

MS disease activity may continue 'below the surface' even when someone is feeling well. Research has shown that, on average, only about one in ten lesions (areas of acute damage) leads to a relapse. In addition, other low-grade tissue damage can also be ongoing. This means that neurological reserve can be depleted even during periods of remission if disease activity is not kept under control.

I really believe that if we – and I mean the entire collegiate of health care professionals who treat MS – can keep the brain health standards at the heart of what we do, the we'll be doing very well for MS patients around the world.

***

An absolute privilege...

I count my fellow MS nurses as amongst my best friends in the world because it's the patterns in our behaviours that draw us to each other. We all experience the same struggles; we all know what we've been through and I daresay we all understand that we can't just walk away from problems or that desire to fix things; to want to make things inherently better. And for as busy as I am and for as many things as I take on in life, I couldn't imagine a time that I'd stop putting my hand up to support my fellow nurses or the organisations that bring us together. But when I do put my hand up to help, I know I'll be supported and that we'll all have each other's back.

Being involved with my patients – often from the very point of their MS diagnosis – is an absolute privilege. To see someone (and their family) on the edge of a cliff as they are digesting the news that their life is going to change irrevocably is intense and it's personal. And I'm invited to share this rollercoaster ride with them and through this I can provide comfort, guidance, and most importantly, hope.

And despite the fact that I might not be an exemplary case study in achieving balance in life, I can manage to find a pretty good sense of perspective. I have devised a multitude of systems so as I can juggle the various assessments and appointments that make up my role. One thing I'd like to do better – and I haven't figured this one out yet – is how to be able to call people back more quickly. If you have any suggestions for that I'd be forever grateful! Most importantly, I start and finish my day with the big picture stuff. My ultimate target is to be able to hand people back their lives; I want my patient to learn how to self-manage. And if I can start and finish the day with that thought – and actually accomplish it along the way – then that's a big tick in my box! When I keep my eyes on that ultimate goal, I can almost (almost!!) allow all the hospital politics to fall into the background.

My little nursing sea change turned out to be one of the best things I've ever done with my life. But once upon a time, I was junior in this field and I recognise it can be very lonely, as most MS nurses work in physical isolation. What a lot of my colleagues may not know about me is that I live with an anxiety disorder; as a teenager I couldn't even talk to someone on the telephone without being a hot, screaming mess, let alone walk into a room and initiate a conversation about something as important as why they are here or stand up in a room of peers to deliver a presentation. And maybe that's why I didn't mind the isolation to a degree. But you know what, despite the hurdles that anxiety presents, I have been able to push through to work with the most amazing, clever, highly motivated group of nurses I have ever known, to contribute to something bigger than me. It's what has fuelled me and together we have been able to contribute to changing the face of MS nursing in Australia.

My hopes for the future treatment and management of MS:

• I hope – and I'm pretty confident – that within the timeframe of my working life, we'll at least find the equivalent of a cure. Treatments are getting so good now and if we can't actually find a way to stop MS from starting then we'll find a preventative measure for future disease.

• And at the same time I can see that we are heading for those that are more targeted towards rebuilding myelin; that we will have a strategy for repair.

• While the most significant advance in treatment in my career has certainly been the development of the disease modifying therapies (DMTs) and the various delivery methods for those, a close second is our approach to MS: seeking timely diagnosis and starting a treatment that will reduce disease is vital to the big picture.

My advice for nurses beginning their career:

• Trust your gut and always put the patient at the heart of your decision. Adopt a mindful approach to MS: pay attention to what is said and, equally, what is not said. Be inquisitive and observant, rather than quick to diagnose and cure.

• Sometimes I've had to advocate for MSers when that runs opposite to what colleagues have planned or suggested, but I feel strongly in these instances those clinicians hadn't heard what the patient had said. Maybe I had more time to listen: either way the outcome was the same.

• The most useful sentence in my vocabulary (and I use it as often as I can) is… 'what can I do for you?' For MSers, well, that's a great way to open a conversation or get it back on track. For setting up new services or trying to squeeze in that extra MSer to a fully booked clinic or service that is at capacity, following up your request with 'and so what I can I do for you?' opens up a dialogue that reflects my understanding they are busy or stretched and maybe there's something I can do to make their job just that little bit easier.

• Try and instil a sense of hope and confidence in your patients. You can't promise them that you can take away the pain or cure the MS but you can promise to be there to talk out their thoughts and develop a plan moving forward and you can promise to try your best to minimise the effects of the MS on their lives.

• Keep reminding your patients that they are not alone. A colleague (and I think my friend), Sally Shaw, developed an analogy that the patient is the CEO of their own MS management company (i.e. their life) and they should recruit the best people to help them run the company: e.g. finance by the person who really knows money, cleaning by, well, not me, ha!. The MS nurse is a director on this board but taking this analogy a little further we can and should help you recruit some of the other specialists you need to have a world-class operation. And if one of these people isn't working to their best for you, time to get a new director in.

• Say yes to every opportunity that comes along. Worry about how you're going to do it later.

• And finally.... hope is everything. If you have lost hope, then you have lost everything. Ensure both you and your patients are carrying hope with them along the journey.

NICOLA 'NICKI' WARD-ABEL
Birmingham, United Kingdom

Becoming a MS nurse is one of the most rewarding jobs in the world because we're at a time that patients can – and are – living with the disease so much better and there's so much we can do to play our part in that.

I grew up in the UK and always wanted to be a nurse and had a very conventional pathway to becoming one. When I turned 18, I did my nurse's training for three years and during that time, several experienced nurses gave me the advice that it was generally better to choose a nursing specialty only after I'd completed quite a few different rotations, allowing me to try my hand at a variety of things. So I started with gastrointestinal before moving into neurology – which I loved – and then went on to become a ward sister in 1989 on the acute neurology ward.

It was here I looked after lots of people with MS, but the people we saw on the wards in those days were not what I would call representative of the MS population we see now. Back then, we were caring for more mature patients, who at that stage of their life had an array of complex health problems. For those early years of my career, I thought that's what MS was. I would often wonder what happened to my patients from the ward once they were discharged. We would spend so much time carefully and lovingly planning for their outpatient care and rehabilitation, but I'd never get to see them again once they were discharged from the hospital, and this saddened me as I love getting to know people.

After a few years of working on the wards, I took some leave to have my first child and when I returned, I found that working on the wards wasn't really what I wanted to do any longer. The schedule didn't suit someone trying to look after a baby and I decided to investigate what other nursing work I might like to do.

Around 1997, the UK introduced a specialist nursing approach to care for people with chronic conditions. The roll out of this specialist nursing concept coincided with more robust drug treatments becoming available for people with MS and clearly there was an opportunity to be at the forefront of this new frontier in nursing.

As a ward sister passionate about patient care but no longer wanting to try and juggle shift work, going into specialist out-patient care seemed ideal and at the same time, quite interesting. In fact, it was a whole new challenge and adventure for me. I thought it would be interesting to learn about the new disease modifying therapies (DMTs) and I could always return to be a ward sister later; but that was twenty years ago and I haven't stopped since!

I 'officially' became a MS nurse in 1997 and about three years later I was approached by the MS Trust. They wanted to know if I'd be willing to take on a new role working half of my time with patients and the rest of my time at Birmingham City University developing and training other nurses who wanted to specialise in multiple sclerosis.

So in 2000, I became the inaugural lecturer of 'The Development of Multiple Sclerosis Care and Management for Specialists' module. It's a week-long residential course for new in-post MS specialist nurses, therapists and other health professionals who specialise in supporting people with MS. The module provides a strong foundation of MS knowledge upon which additional specialist knowledge can develop, and covers a host of clinical and professional issues relevant to health care providers undertaking a specialist role.

It was a wonderful opportunity because I could continue working with my patients in the MS service I'd established in Birmingham and also play a role in developing the nurses of tomorrow. By this stage I already knew I loved teaching and I'd become such an advocate on the power of education, so it really was the best of both worlds.

I started off teaching nurses and therapists who wanted to specialise in multiple sclerosis and then I would also provide more comprehensive skills to nurses in the community who were caring for patients with complex needs, including – but not limited to – MS. After a few years, the role developed into teaching student nurses as well, ensuring they had a minimum of ten hours dedicated to learning about MS as part of their wider nursing degree. I'm not aware that any other university in the UK was offering this type of module at the time and it was serendipitous that I worked at the Birmingham clinic and could develop the course.

Most nurses tend to find their specialisation by default and learn on the job. The vision of the MS Trust was far different in that it wanted to ensure that MS specialist nurses were offered a great deal more education from the onset. Since the inception of this foundation course, the MS Trust has committed to offering a fixed number of fully funded places to those working in a MS specialist nurse's role. The course remains fully accredited by the university as counting towards a bachelor or master's degree and approximately forty nurses a year undertake the course and go on to work in multiple sclerosis, as well as other neurological conditions.

***

I think the formalisation of MS nursing has revolutionised patient care in MS.

There was a while there in the UK that people with MS were definitely considered the unpopular type of patients; there was this misconception that they were demanding and difficult.

I think perhaps the misconception developed in a time when we didn't have enough experienced MS nurses who could dedicate and provide a continuity of care to people living with the disease. A decade ago, a patient would have gone to the hospital for a check-up or visited a clinic with a doctor or nurse they'd never met before and then probably had everything about their care changed around. I'd hear about this process going on time-after-time when they met a new health care professional. It's little wonder a person with MS might get a bit cranky if their care was constantly in flux! People with MS tend to work out for themselves how they need to be cared for and I think as doctors and nurses, we don't listen enough to the patient's input.

In my classes, I needed to demonstrate that the perception of the 'difficult and demanding' MS patient was all wrong. Now – with proper care and attention – we are seeing people who are living very well with MS. I want to instil in my students that becoming a MS nurse is one of the most rewarding jobs in the world because we're at a time that patients can and are living with the disease so much better and there's so much we can do to play our part in that.

When I first started out as a MS nurse, there was only about eight of us in the entire country. Our MS patients would just embrace our work (and us as people) so warmly. I think it was because they finally had someone who would sit and listen to them and take the time to understand. It's one thing for a person living with MS to have great family and friends to give them support, but that support network can fall into its own fatigue and can't always be there, and sometimes that support network simply doesn't know what sort of help to give. As nurses, we offer a different perspective and a different form of support entirely. To that extent, I think the formalisation of MS nursing has revolutionised patient care in MS. We're able to fill a big gap between the GP and the family and now, all these years later, combine forces with the neurologists to offer a really top-notch level of support.

What also needs to be recognised is that there are many, many things that a person with MS will feel more comfortable talking to their MS nurse about but won't even touch the same topic with their GP, neurologist or family and friends. And these can be serious problems, which may be left completely unrecognised and unattended if it weren't for our role in the patient's care. MS nurses are now being trained to recognise the types of problems that a patient might be reticent to tackle: The patient will delicately tread around the issue but the nurses will be able to rephrase the concern and raise it with their patients in such a way that they'll feel more comfortable speaking about it. They'll create a connection that allows a patient to feel secure with the nurse's empathy, but also find the touchpoints that will hopefully resonate enough for them to be open to assistance or advice.

The continuity in care these days has changed so much that patients are still surprised when I can remember their names and personally greet them in the waiting room! We don't remember everything about everyone, but we do take a great interest in their life as a whole – because so many lifestyle factors will influence their health outcomes – and we start to build up a history with them. I joke with some of my patients that we're growing old together and that they probably know as much about my life as I do theirs! I have to clarify though, that I don't consider myself to be there to be my patient's friend; that would be inappropriate. However, we are definitely seen as compassionate people who know them well, and in many cases, know more about certain parts of their life than a friend might.

I think a good MS nurse will be able to determine when a patient needs you to give medical and health advice and when they just need you to listen. Even the act of talking about a problem can tremendously unburden a patient. A friend, however, will nearly always want to give advice, and that's not always necessary or even the best solution.

The simple tonic of allowing someone to talk while we sit and listen is so underrated. I want my patients to tell it how it is and just let them get things off their chest. I don't need to be constantly jumping into their 'unburdening,' feeling like every little detail needs to be dissected or fixed. There are those times the patient just needs to rant and unload and divest themselves of the concern so as they can get it off their mind.

Having said that, if one of my patients tells me about a health problem that I know we can improve or even fix, then I will very patiently and carefully listen to everything they're saying but then I'll absolutely come in at the end and do my best to problem solve something that I think we have a good chance of fixing. After more than twenty years as a MS nurse, I know the better tactic to problem solving things with a patient is to listen and then listen some more and then offer 'suggestions' at the end. It might be a very gentle process of drip-feeding suggestions or ideas. Basically building on the information bit by bit, particularly when we're discussing solutions or treatments that are huge and life changing. A good MS nurse will be able to gauge their patient and make a judgement call on how much information they want or can take on at any given point in time. And you can only do all of that from experience.

One of my biggest challenges is time management. And I fear that this far into my career I'm never going to learn! But one technique I employ in consultations is to ask my patients to think of (or come prepared with) three main things they need to talk to me about on the day. I will actually sit with my patient and write those three things out, so we can focus on their particular areas of concern. I also find that by writing the things down together, we push all other distractions away and that in itself alleviates stress.

There was a survey done in the UK only a few years back and it found that for every clinic visit, on average a patient would raise eight different things. And if you did a home visit, then that number expanded out to thirteen issues raised with the nurse. You just can't get through all of that. It's terrible to admit, but you just can't! If it were up to me to schedule two hours with every patient, I'd do it in a heartbeat. But we have other conflicting interests at play. The NHS needs us to see more patients yet keep our clinics running on time and of course, we have nursing duties outside of patient consultations that need attending to. There really isn't enough time to do it all! So my 'three main things' rule is very handy. It doesn't always go according to plan; it doesn't always keep people focussed and sometimes I'll need to gently suggest we address the 'just one more thing' topic at the next appointment, but if I can at least try to keep people focussed then we all (sort of) win.

***

In many ways, the content of patient consultations really hasn't changed too much over the last two decades, particularly for the newly diagnosed. They always ask 'the wheelchair' question; that is – the vast majority want to know – "will I end up in a wheelchair?" And over time I've come to challenge my patients a bit over that outlook. I try to clarify why some people with MS are in wheelchairs and others are not. I want them to understand that MS is very individualised for everyone. Some people are in wheelchairs as they're experiencing a relapse at that point in time, others just need to use a chair to get from A to B to conserve energy, and others still may have been living with MS for decades and not had access to the more efficacious treatments we have today.

I also find that those newly diagnosed today want a game plan more immediately. They want to know what we're going to do about the MS and when they can start on a treatment. Whereas twenty years ago, someone with MS may have waited a long, long time to be diagnosed and may not have even gone onto a treatment. Over the last few years I have noticed a very strong sense of urgency for the newly diagnosed to focus on the drug treatments up front.

And in a way, I find the dogged focus on drugs a bit of a problem. In no way do I want to take away from the fact that people newly diagnosed with MS today have access to DMTs that have shown great promise at halting the disease and allowing people to live pretty full lives. We also know that about 25 percent of people diagnosed with MS in the UK are on the newer DMTs that require stricter monitoring and thus regularly see a health care professional to oversee the treatment; but what about the other 75% of people with MS? I find it hard to reconcile that just because a patient isn't on one of the newer DMTs – let alone those people who can't or don't take a treatment – are not getting the same frequency and perhaps continuity of care that a patient on the newer DMTs would. So many of our clinics are now more about managing the drugs and unfortunately that means we put the non DMT-patients on a once-a-year visit. It's just not enough. I'm passionate about campaigning for a change in this.

As I mentioned, one of my most frustrating challenges is there simply isn't enough time to do everything I want to for my patients. And then we marry this up with the fact there's only so much that we can 'actually' do for our patients as well. We sort of created a rod for our backs when we set about to fill in the gaps of personalised care that a neurologist might not have been able to provide. I know anecdotally our patients feel they need to be very brief and business-like with their neurologists. They would feel like they were only allocated five precious minutes, so they better get in, be direct and move on. Whereas the relationship we tend to cultivate with our patients as MS nurses is more one of approachability and allowing our patients the time and a safe environment to ask the things they didn't feel comfortable asking their neurologist. And of course, we've made ourselves more accessible than the neurologist as well, so it's hardly surprising that we find ourselves full to the brim with patient enquiries and responsibilities. I just find it devastating that I can't give more time to those patients who really need it.

At our clinic, we give our patients a thirty-minute consultation. We know we could probably cover everything in about twenty minutes but then you miss out of the subtleties of indulging the patient with some gentle small talk. And this small talk often uncovers other niggling issues that have been masked by the 'big stuff,' or vice versa. Those extra few minutes allow me to ask about the family or support network. Or if my patient has brought a family member or partner, it allows me to ask the family member how they think their loved one is going. A great deal of information can be unveiled through these seemingly innocent conversations.

I also find it frustrating that too many patients I see have missed the opportunity altogether of being able to get onto a treatment that may help them. It's generally those people who find themselves with progressive MS and for one reason or another they haven't been able to take a medication to try and keep the MS at bay. They find themselves with deteriorating symptoms and they are desperate and pleading for the opportunity to take something that may help. They are literally happy to be human guinea pigs and weather the risk of taking a DMT or other treatment that we know won't help them. Of course we can't allow it, and we have to work hard to have them understand that we aren't withholding drugs – or hope – but that we just can't ethically allow people to start on a drug that isn't approved for their stage of MS. But having those people sitting in front of me, begging for help, is one of the most heart-breaking things I see.

At the other end of the spectrum is the treatment of adolescents with MS. As MS nurses, we're very well versed to treat adults but treating teenagers is a whole other thing. There's just so many psychological challenges we have to navigate with the young patients and we don't have a lot of learnings and case studies to draw from. We're getting better at it, although we still have so much to learn.

But I think the thing I struggle with the most is when my patients are also experiencing co-morbidities and psychiatric issues. You can just see everything feeding into a big rolling snow ball. And then if the parents or partners are also feeling that stress, it often manifests in their questioning of my ability to manage the situation suitably. In those times – where everyone concerned might be at the end of their tether – I might be confronted with a frustrated family member asking why I'm not doing more? They may feel my full attention is not being given to their loved one. I totally understand the frustration and at the same time, I've still got to juggle a thousand things competing for my attention on any given day.

Hearing about relationship breakdowns in the lives' of my patients with MS is the other thing I find challenging. Not only is there the heartbreak of losing a partner, but I can see the inherent fear a patient is feeling when they realise they may have to manage this disease alone. My heart really goes out to those people.

Unfortunately, I know there's no easy fix to any of these frustrations. We just have to work smarter; look at ways we can transfer some responsibilities to free up our time for patients. Maybe have the pharmaceutical company nurses manage some of the patient education tasks? Certainly, we need to keep sharing information amongst our colleagues. We're pretty good at doing this and so many of our MS nurses around the world are passionate about seeing the continual and evolving sharing of stories and skills. I also think technology is going to help us greatly in the not-too-distant future. I think someone, at some stage, will create the perfect app that a patient can use to share information with their health care team and to monitor symptoms and aspects of their disease. Imagine a situation where a MS nurse could quickly download their patient's vital data from an app prior to their consultation, skim over the data and possibly save time because they didn't have to ask a lot of basic questions to play catch up? Technology may serve a role in helping us prioritise issues within the consultation or by providing a more accurate way of recording information so patients didn't need to rely as much on memorising or recalling lots of details.

***

Education is power.

My career has given me the opportunity to travel the world, something I could never have imagined when I was just starting out in nursing. In fact, I remember the first ever conference I was invited to. It was only about six months after becoming a MS nurse and a colleague mentioned that there was a spare place to attend an upcoming workshop in Istanbul. My immediate and extremely shy response was 'oh gosh... I don't think I'd be allowed!' But I nervously rang my supervisor anyway, thinking I should at least get his response so I could rule the opportunity out. Well, to my surprise, he was a bit incredulous I was calling to ask permission and actually sounded like I was wasting his time. He merely said "Don't be silly. Of course you can go." It was as simple as that!

We are blessed in our MS community that sharing information, developing our professional knowledge and learning from each other around the globe has always been highly regarded and prioritised. We all think we're very clever in the countries in which we work and we all think we've got it sorted, but then we all get together as international colleagues and we hear each other's ideas and processes and problems, and we go on to learn brilliant things.

From a personal point of view though, I could never have imagined that I would stand on a stage in front of hundreds of people in another country and talk to them about MS. I have been afforded so many amazing opportunities to speak about something I'm passionate about.

And once you start putting yourself out there, you start developing other connections and friends and the opportunities continue to expand. I'm so grateful to have been invited onto working groups that have allowed me to not only feed my passion but continue building my own working knowledge. I'm currently involved in a project called MS Nurse Professional *(msnursepro.org)* that allows MS nurses all over Europe to share their knowledge with other nurses online. Every time we launch in a new country we ensure everything is fully translated and we can accredit the information shared into professional development points for the MS nurses. In the UK we have education coming out of our ears but there are some regions in Europe which are not as lucky. We all nurse very differently and have to do so within the confines of a variety of health care systems. Education is power.

And one of the best ways we can continue truly supporting our patients is if we are educated to our highest potential with the most up-to-date information.

Sexual wellbeing in people with MS has always been a specialty area for me and I've been lucky enough to present on the topic around the world. It's also created one of the worst situations that I didn't quite know how to fix! A few years back, I decided it would be good to run little mini workshops at the clinic for my patients about MS and sexual health. Well, we had a good attendance and patients brought their partners and the discussions were quite open and easy going. Then suddenly the vibe in the group turned and I had couples pointing the finger at each other in accusation of not doing this or not doing that and basically pandemonium just erupted amongst everyone airing their sexual frustrations. I eventually got everyone to calm down but I decided the group sessions probably weren't such a good idea and I had learned a valuable lesson that I was NOT a relationship counsellor!

I think as MS nurses we try to do too much. We want to go that extra mile for our patients and their families, but we should probably rein ourselves in on a great many things; we should learn what our boundaries are. You just have to cultivate a good sense of knowing when to pass an issue onto someone who's better equipped to deal with it.

I know that many of my colleagues and fellow MS nurses have different strategies for putting everything they see and do in perspective – particularly the heartbreaking stuff – but I just don't think I do. I tend to just sit and cry alongside my patients when I hear about the terrible stuff. Often, I have no solution, (let alone any right) to try and fix what they're going through, so sometimes all I can do is hold their hand and cry with them.

But can I separate myself from my patient's grief? Yes, I think so. I have a theory that my uniform is representative of the line between nurse and patient. It allows me to listen and be empathetic and certainly feel everything I need to feel. But my uniform is also representative of the type of role I play in my patient's life and no matter how touched I am by my patients, I know the uniform gives me permission to go home at night and not carry their grief with me.

Most patients at some point go into complete catastrophisation mode. A lot of my role as a MS nurse is to question their beliefs as to what they think will happen with the MS and then steer their thought patterns into one of rationality and perspective. I find I'll often have to dig deep to unravel what they believe is going to happen – not necessarily what IS happening at that point – and then re-shape their perspective by way of educating with fact and research. We talk in terms of probability and also timeframes. Some of the things my patients are fearful of, may happen in the future, but it's not happening now; and as such, those fears shouldn't be allowed to control your life now. I would just hate to see any of my patients spending their life worrying about something that may never happen. It's a life half lived.

I also like to teach mindfulness techniques; I think an attitude of calm acceptance can be good for a great many people in any situation, but I believe people living with a chronic illness can benefit from learning to live without the judgement that there's a right or wrong way to feel in any given moment. And mindset is such an important part of anyone's disease course management. Mindset and attitude have nothing to do with the DMTs but everything to do with how that person wants to prevail over this disease; how they want to find joy or meaning or fulfillment in their life rather than misery and hopelessness and loneliness.

Lifestyle factors are also hugely important for me to assist my patients getting their mind around. It's part of cultivating their 'take control' mindset in fact. We didn't talk a lot about lifestyle factors for a long time but now we know how important it is to take a holistic approach to managing MS. It's about a healthy diet and getting exercise and managing your energy wisely, not smoking and getting plenty of vitamin D; all the sustainable lifestyle factors to promote good brain and body health. I think it's really empowering for anyone living with MS to be able to take control of the lifestyle factors themselves.

I've been a MS nurse for over twenty years and although I couldn't be more passionate about my profession, I never thought I'd been doing this job for as long as I have. And while I love the teaching, it's the patients that mean the most to me. The simplest but most profound gratification I get is when a patient confides to me, "you know what, I did what you suggested, and it made such a difference. I feel a lot better." It's the best feeling in the world to think something you did might have helped someone. I really mean it.

**

Author's Note

Nicki sadly passed away in September 2018 after a courageous battle with cancer. I feel truly blessed that I was able to interview her for this book in April of that year. She was an inspiration to all who knew her, always showing courage and determination to not give in, and she has left a gaping hole in the hearts of her colleagues and the nursing world.

My hopes for the future treatment and management of MS:

• When I started, we had two drug treatments we could give out, and now we have fourteen. The way that we can now address a patient's MS at relapse number one is just unbelievably good news to me. I truly believe we're changing the natural history of their disease by the fact that we can treat so much more effectively and so much earlier. Fancy being able to do that!! Compared to what MS could have been for some people, imagine being able to create a better outcome!!

• I think if we can achieve a situation where MS is no longer the first thing a patient thinks of in the morning when they wake up, then that's amazing in itself too.

• I'd love to come back in a hundred years and see what the really smart people figured out about how MS is caused. I sort of think that they'd be laughing at what we thought might cause MS and what actually does. I believe once we know what causes MS, the treatments and repair and all the other stuff will follow very quickly.

• I'm also wishing with every fibre of my body that we could make things better for people with progressive MS.

My advice for nurses beginning their career:

• Work hard and play hard! We work really hard and you need to work out how to balance that by finding joy and fun in life.

• Make sure you always have time for yourself. You may want to change the world and make your patient's life better, but you can't do that without taking time for yourself to nurture or recharge the batteries.

• Read, read and then read some more. There are so many great resources available now to keep up-to-date on everything to do with MS and healthy lifestyles.

• If you're a MS nurse working on your own, make sure you reach out to other MS nurses somehow, whether it's attending workshops and conferences or participating in online forums.

• Preparatory work is also key. If you're settling into a new job or starting a new clinic, try and build in some time initially where you don't see any patients at all. I know it sounds like a complete luxury, but if you had a bit of time to yourself to set up your systems and get to know your database of patients and even organise the way that allows you to work more efficiently from the beginning, you will reap the rewards. Because let's face it.... once you start the job, you won't be able to stop and take a break to recalibrate systems.

KAREN VERNON
Greater Manchester, United Kingdom

*If there's one word that I can use to describe my career, it's 'fortunate.'
Being a MS nurse has allowed me opportunities I could never have
imagined, and to develop friendships unlike any I've ever experienced.*

....

I don't know what it is, but there's a really special sense of
comradery that we experience as MS nurses. It's one that
stretches across the globe. And I know just how unique and special
it is, because other colleagues in different specialties often remark
how they've never experienced anything quite like the international
bonds we share as MS nurses. And I can't put my finger on whether
it's because of the types of personalities who are drawn to this role as
a MS nurse or whether it's in fact the patients who bind us together.
Or maybe it's the outstanding opportunities we have to regularly
come together as MS specialty nurses and share our experiences.

***

I've been nursing since I was 18, and in neurology since 1985. In
fact, my experience in neurology nursing far outdates the availability
of the disease modifying treatments (DMTs) for Multiple Sclerosis.
I began my career working within the acute neuro wards as a ward
nurse before going on to become the unit manager. And it was in
the position as the unit manager that I started appointing special-

ist nurses into their roles. In fact, I was instrumental in appointing the first ever specialist MS nurse into her role during the introduction of the betaferon treatments. The appointment of a specialist Parkinson's Disease nurse was to follow, and I guess that's when I really started to take notice of the very unique attributes these nurses were bringing to their patients: It fascinated me. Around the same time, a supervisor of mine was urging me to get out of my comfort zone and pursue a new role that had just come up; one that would allow me to push myself more and gain some new insights. It was further afield than where I was living but this role as a community neurology nurse was too intriguing to pass up.

The post as a community neurology nurse involved caring for people not only with Multiple Sclerosis but also Parkinson's Disease and Motor Neurone Disease. The DMTs had just started to change the practice of MS nursing and the timing would open the door to be part of what would be a monumental change in the treatment and care of MS and I could already envision the difference that specialist nursing in this field could make. I think I knew fundamentally that being a specialist nurse would give me the ability to care holistically for someone.

During this time I also undertook a post-graduate diploma in the ethics of cancer and palliative care. It may seem like an odd thing to study whilst I was fully immersed in the neurology track, but I wanted to ensure I had a wide range of skills that made me employable in a number of situations. And once I was studying the diploma, I realised how applicable it was to my neuro patients. The diploma was actually a mix of disciplines and specialties and was also culturally diverse. I gained so much knowledge through this course; it really demonstrated to me the value of striving for the best interests of my patients and always ensuring I had the patient at the heart of what I needed to do. It's very much a practice I've taken into my career as a MS nurse and still something I coach the student nurses about today.

I'm also not afraid to talk to people about dying and again, it's a useful skill to have when dealing with MS patients. I find I can have frank and open discussions with my patients, especially those who express a fear of death and MS. I can drop little nuggets of information and they'll come to realise they're not going to die from MS but they will die 'with' it. Often their fear stems from the aspect of dying – understandably – but has nothing at all to do with having MS. I think through studying palliative care I've developed skills that allow me to initiate difficult conversations and ask the hard questions, not only about death but really across a very broad range of topics and to a wide variety of patients, family members and carers.

I remained in the community nurse role for six years and by that stage, I was firmly committed to furthering my career within MS. So I set about obtaining the qualification to become a MS Specialist Nurse and then added to this with the credentials of a Multiple Sclerosis Nurse Consultant.

Salford Hospital in Manchester was one of the first hospitals to develop the role of the MS Nurse Consultant. The neurologists saw this as a senior nursing role, where a highly qualified nurse could be brought in to assess the patient. And whilst the role was initially developed because of the introduction of DMTs, the MS Nurse Consultant became well-utilised in a general clinical sense as there simply wasn't enough capacity in the clinics for the neurologists to see all the patients. The role was fifty percent clinical consultations – or supervision of the consultations – and the other fifty percent was managerial with a dash of research responsibility thrown in along with education and teaching. It's quite a broad set of responsibilities and I also have a large geographical area to cover.

The service covers the whole of Greater Manchester and east Cheshire and we have a combined MS population of 4,700 patients, who are officially known to the service, with an estimated further 300 patients who are not officially registered. We are the tertiary prescribing centre and have approximately 1,700 patients approved by the NHS England to be taking a DMT but we work with patients from across the whole of the disease trajectory.

***

In March 2012, the UK Trust published a ground-breaking report titled Defining the value of MS specialist nurses. This report would be the first integral piece in what would go on to become the 'Generating Evidence for MS Services' project, or GEMSS for short.

The GEMSS report identified that whilst people with MS and other health professionals had a compelling story to tell about the positive value of MS specialist nurses, there was little robust published evidence about their value and effectiveness. The majority of MS nurses were not routinely evaluating their services due to a lack of time, skills and tools to do so.

So to capture this important evidence, in 2012 the MS Trust launched the GEMSS Programme and began working with MS nurses to co-develop an evaluation framework and a set of tools and metrics for services. The aims of the project were to build the skills and capabilities of the nurses, while developing a culture of continuous improvement.

The GEMSS work has now expanded beyond MS specialist nurses and the tools developed as part of the programme have been adapted for use by any MS team, including Allied Health Professionals with a special interest in MS.

The MS Trust used early outputs from the GEMSS evaluation projects to develop a consensus report called 'Modelling Sustainable Caseloads: MS Specialist Nurses,' which identified a sustainable caseload for a MS specialist nurse and also the conditions that needed to be present for the service to be effective within that caseload. Subsequently, the UK Trust were able to map the current UK workforce against this benchmark.

I was involved in the GEMSS project from the beginning as the lead for the Salford Royal NHS Foundation Trust.

The GEMSS project has revolutionised our service and allowed us to secure more nursing positions because of this research. Within my service, we now have the equivalent of 5.8 full time senior MS nurses and 2.8 support nurses along with two administration and support workers. My team organise themselves based on geographical areas across Manchester but in general, each nurse is managing a caseload of around 800 patients, which I would suggest is completely unsustainable. They do, on average, three clinics per week across the area but invariably the monitoring requirements are taking over the clinic slots and those patients who are not taking a DMT are losing out.

I find it quite alarming to review the data on the increasing number of patients that we now only see every twelve months or less. I think we actually need a team within a team: A team of nurses who are dedicated to seeing the non-DMT patients and focus on complex symptom management and progressive MS. Ensuring that the non-DMT patients are getting an appropriate level of care in our DMT environment is something I feel a strong sense of legacy in creating before I retire.

The GEMSS programme provided everyone with a lot of food for thought; not only in the UK but also our MS Specialist Nursing collegiate internationally. It very much reinforced the importance of a multidisciplinary service to comprehensively meet the needs of people with MS. None of the health or social care professionals who work with people affected by MS can be effective in isolation.

GEMSS provided me with many insights and also time to pause and think about what an ideal team would look like. In a perfect world, I think the team would be led by an experienced nurse possessing a breadth of skills across neurology, neurological rehab and even oncology. And then of course the team would mentor some more junior nurses who are willing to learn and would definitely include therapists and administrative support resources.

And if I could be really, really specific, I'd ideally recruit nurses who learned their craft through MS symptom management and I'd then upskill those nurses into treatment management rather than the other way around. I think there's a lot of nurses being put into treatment management posts and whilst they are excellent nurses, they lack the hands-on experience at dealing with symptom management.

In examining our resources and capabilities, my mind has also turned to succession planning for the sustainability of not only our service but also our profession. In the UK there's more nurses leaving the NHS system than ever before. We're seeing highly trained nurses leaving and retiring; they just want to find a better lifestyle than what being a NHS-system nurse can offer them. Then on the other end of the scale, we know that in recent years there's been some 10,000 less applications annually for students wanting to enter nursing at university. The Universities and Colleges Admissions Service (UCAS) reported that the number of nursing applicants in England had fallen by a pretty staggering 23% over the last few years. There were 43,800 applicants in January 2016 and just 33,810 in January

2017 and the 2018 figures were on track for a 12% decrease in applications to enter nursing.

I'm just not sure where we're going to get new nurses from or how we're going to keep our current nursing colleagues engaged in the system. Brexit will further effect things and certainly add a number of hoops to jump through. We're very lucky in MS nursing that we rarely have too many vacancies and we tend to attract good candidates because of the many educational and professional opportunities that the role brings. But as a MS community, we've had to work hard at building these opportunities and this good reputation and I don't think for a moment we can be complacent. Due to the ever-changing nature of both the MS treatment landscape and the health system, we always need to be looking at how we can be managing the processes whilst also simultaneously driving improvements.

***

Frustrations…. I've got a few!

I think the people living with progressive MS get a bit of a raw deal and it continues to be one of my biggest frustrations. They aren't given time for the clinic appointments as frequently as someone being monitored on a DMT and as a MS service, the number of home visit consultations we're able to facilitate has dropped dramatically as well. Unfortunately we just find ourselves in a health system that is trying to squeeze as much productivity and value out of everything they can and clinics are seen as being far more efficient and financially viable than home visits.

And I understand that many people with progressive MS get to a point where they become disengaged with the MS service, but it's a vicious circle, because if we can't see these patients, then we don't know that they're unhappy or feeling neglected and it becomes a difficult problem to fix. I know there's a great deal of angst amongst the cohort of patients who miss out on the care and symptom management just because they were unable to take a treatment in the first place.

And it's understandable, because they'll see great innovation in the treatment of MS but this in turn brings disappointment and anxiety about their own situation. The area of stem cell treatments is always a hotbed for us. Autologous haematopoietic stem cell transplant (AHSCT) is a very tricky treatment to explain and yet the media always latch onto it, launching a flurry of enquiries to our MS service, often from the people who frustratingly feel like they've run out of options. And we have no choice but to tell the truth that AHSCT is simply not a treatment that is any way suitable for a patient living with progressive MS.

The difference in providing symptom management processes in something like cancer compared to MS also confounds me. When someone is being treated for cancer, the education and prioritisation of symptom management is seen as a positive. In the long run, it's considered good for patients and the health care system alike. It's supported and encouraged by the health care professionals and in turn, the patients are far more likely to be better attuned to symptom management. But in MS, I'm often left with the feeling that symptom management is just an option – and even carries slightly negative connotations – for patients.

I'm constantly talking to the nurses to create a level playing field between treatment selection and its monitoring, alongside the symptom management; explaining that no matter how good the DMT is, a patient will still need to maintain their own health and wellbeing and manage their symptoms. We know how beneficial it is for a person newly diagnosed with MS to find a suitable treatment as soon after diagnosis as possible and I see how much better these people do on treatment, but I think whilst treatment options are the big focus in those early months we're missing a very important window of opportunity to get the patient and their family to understand so many other things about MS. They often won't understand the commitment to these aggressive treatments, they won't understand the modifiable lifestyle factors that may help and they may not fully comprehend the range of symptoms that could manifest and how to manage those.

As part of NHS England recommendations when prescribing a DMT, we now have a multi-disciplinary team (MDT) that will discuss patient cases to ensure eligibility and consistency of approach is used. The team currently consists of the consultants, nurses, co-ordinators and in the future a neuro pharmacist.

Concerns might include whether the treatment delivery method is a good fit in terms of compliancy for the patient and if the monitoring process could be adhered to. It's often the nurses who bring some of the 'home truths' to the table as we generally have a better feel for the patient's ability to manage treatments because of their social situation. We may need to consider their living arrangements, such as whether they're living in a disadvantaged environment or are in fact homeless, both of which are quite common in the greater Manchester area. In these cases, we might suggest that a 28-day infusion is a better option; we feel that turning up to the clinic once a month might be more manageable and that the patient could get a little TLC at the same time. This is not a criticism of the neurologists, but I have found that patients tend to explain the non-medical aspects of their lives with greater ease to the nurse.

Frankly, these roundtable multi-disciplinary meetings can be quite eye opening for all involved and I think when we have five different neurologists who all practice in a variety of ways, these roundtables are essential so as we can bring some cohesion and clinical governance approach to our service. I can also see that in the future we'll be able to bring all complex patient cases into the multi-disciplinary meetings – whether they're on a treatment or not.

***

The task of managing MS falls on the shoulders of many people.

One of the most common questions someone newly diagnosed with MS will ask me is simply 'what will happen?' It can be so hard to explain the inevitable frustration they are likely to experience and more so because there are very few 'yes' or 'no' answers in multiple sclerosis. As nurses, we find ourselves frequently talking in terms of 'this might happen' and 'that might happen' but we just can't always give definitives. I fully understand how exasperating that must be for people living with MS. As nurses, we have to be very careful to put everything into context for the individual patient and this may mean using a variety of different communication styles. We have lots of research and studies to draw information and statistics from and similarly, our breadth of experience can also give us a lot of different anecdotes and case studies to represent a point. It's about being truthful but balancing that truth with hope and realism of what living with this disease can be like. Shaping the mindset of the newly diagnosed in those early years is really crucial for their outlook and acceptance.

I also believe that general health and well-being is really important for the newly diagnosed to continue embracing. It can't all just be about 'the MS' and as we know, poor health can feed into the MS creating a big snowball effect. And strong and stable mental health is absolutely crucial, especially given that we have evidence that depression and anxiety is more prevalent in people living with MS.

And patients continue to ask questions about life expectancy and MS – even today with all the literature out there – and how I would answer is that none of us really know what our life expectancy is... It may not sound like the happiest response but my consultation style over the years has evolved quite a bit to become more honest and pragmatic. Especially in a time where we're often trying to play catch up in providing good generalised information about living with MS after a patient has been focussed on the DMT side of things in those early days.

The task of managing MS falls on the shoulders of many people – not just the person diagnosed with the disease – but also obviously their family, the specialist neurologists and nurses, and also allied health professionals and health care providers. But it's a big cast of people to manage and it often comes down to the nurses to try and coordinate all of these people. But therein lies another frustration. Some health care systems – such as ours in the UK – just don't provide for enough specialist help and so many people too often fall between the cracks. Even if we are in a timely position to see a patient during a relapse and make a referral to a specialist such as a physiotherapist or occupational therapist, then it may be many months before the patient can secure a consultation with that specialist and then many more months before we see the patient again to review the recommendations of the other health professional. There just seem to be so many missed windows of opportunity to provide the best continuity of care that we know we're capable of.

And on the flip side of this story are the specialists who provide therapies for people with progressive MS. Now I've already discussed how as nurses we don't generally get to see the progressive patients more than once a year. But there's a knock-on effect to that. If we're not seeing these patients as often, then we're unable to refer them out for treatments and services to specialists in this area of progressive MS and then those specialists become disengaged as well and everyone misses out on the benefit of this expert advice.

More and more I see progressive MS as an area that is largely self-managed by the patient and unfortunately, it's at a time they generally could do with more assistance.

As nurses, we all have to accept that people will make choices that they feel are right for them at that point in time – no matter how much information we give them. And sadly, sometimes those choices are going to be bad choices. Occasionally we're lucky enough to wear people down and get them to do something we believe is in their best interest! But by and large, a patient just has to be at the right place and the right time to accept things and go on to fully embrace it. I don't believe that people deliberately bury their head in the sand. I just believe it's a way that some people cope with things and process information in the short term. And there's nearly always reasons why people do things the way they do, be it having issues with compliance or similar – they're not obstinate or stubborn – but my feeling is that those people who have issues time and again are the patients who just haven't understood from the beginning the importance of what has to happen and the impact that their actions will have on their own health. It can be a big learning curve for the patient, but also us as nurses.

There are just so many details to take on at the time of diagnosis (and all throughout the MS journey if I was being honest) and it's so immensely overwhelming. But as nurses we have to keep plugging away at delivering information and ensuring our patients are taking on what they can, when they can. We rarely experience instant gratification in this job. Instead I find it a thrill when patients will approach me many years later and confide a win or a lifestyle change they made. They'll often say things like "do you remember way back when you told me to do x,y,z? Well, I finally did it and now I feel much better," or "I managed to be able to do this, this and that." Those small wins are still very gratifying for me, no matter when and where they materialise from.

***

Keeping everything in perspective.

It doesn't matter how long I've been in this job – I still find there are constantly things that I don't know how to fix. And often I have to stand back to figure out the situation for what it is, but also contemplate if I'm even the best person to fix whatever is wrong. Then there's other things that are just so terribly hard to fix – or are perhaps unfixable – and we have to be realistic and understand that they may be beyond our control. In these times, I like to reflect on what we could learn from this situation? In my recent career, I've attended some case discussions (one of which was fatal) of progressive multifocal leukoencephalopathy (PML), caused by biological therapies that allow JC virus reactivation. It's just a devastating situation for everyone involved and it's obviously something that stays with you for a long time. But I counsel my team to ensure they learn from everything they possibly can.

It can be difficult to keep the big picture in front of you, particularly if you're constantly putting out lots of little fires. Some of those pressure points might occur in times when I have staff away sick or new staff transitioning into the service. It's important we look after ourselves in order to look after others.

It's still important to divide my attention between both the large and small issues, especially in my job; because I have to know what's going on but I still need to be in a position to insightfully drive things forward.

I guess time management is at the heart of what I struggle with the most. And that's not to say I mismanage time but more the fact that I have so much that needs to be achieved within a very limited amount of time. And looking after my own personal wellbeing often

TAKING CONTROL COMPASSIONATELY

gets pushed to the end of the line in this equation.

I look after my team extremely well, but that's curiously also part of the problem. Recently when I stood back and pondered the situation, I recognised that too frequently I'd step in to help other members of the team. They were under similar time constraints and I simply didn't want time management issues to unravel and impact the rest of the team as a whole. I felt that assisting my team in picking up the slack was part of my role but what I'd overlooked is it's actually a trait of a strong team dynamic for the entire team to pull in together themselves. And it's certainly more sustainable to try and rally together rather than carry the problem single-handedly. But it remains a hard thing to reconcile in yourself, because as a manager, you want your team - and the service you provide to patients - to be an all-star experience. But you could easily burn yourself out trying to achieve this by carrying the load by yourself. My personal outlook on this now, is to try and take a longer term and measured approach to everything, rather than running around trying to apply a quick fix. Easier said than done!

We also have a very strong clinical governance structure where I work, and this assists my management processes enormously. It means that every other month I can bring the entire team together to talk through compliance, complaints, risks, policy and protocol and for everyone to offer their feedback or advice.

Finding a way to keep everything in perspective is just so important. There is sadness in what we do and as nurses we deal with some very difficult and confronting situations. MS is a disease that can have a nasty habit of sneaking up on you and reminding you how bloody horrible it can be. And it always takes you by surprise. Every single time.

I'm careful to look after my team in these situations, and without sounding flippant, I find humour gets us through a lot of things. And maybe it's also the humour that allows us to open up to each other on the team and provide the support needed. But just as importantly, as a manager it's paramount that I recognise when a team member needs a kind of support we can't offer to one another and perhaps counselling or resilience training in a different environment is a better solution.

***

We attract all types!

I don't see the level of burn out amongst specialist MS nurses as I do in some other nursing areas. And on the very rare occasions I do see it, the common factor has been a lack of engagement with the MS community, so I truly believe that the connectiveness to both the patients (for engagement) and their MS nursing colleagues (for 'networking' and mutual support) is very important.

And I don't subscribe to a certain personality type being attracted to MS nursing, (as we attract all types!) but I do think that because most MS nurses have seen the landscape of their professional development grow in tandem with the increasing research into MS as a disease – and the ensuing development of treatments – we all unite together to protect and nurture the environment in which we passionately operate. And by that very nature, we also nurture one-another.

Being able to stay in my specialty for as long as I have and see this growth and transition within clinical nursing has been one of the most brilliant things about my career. And I think our entire MS nursing community would feel privileged to be in a speciality where we've seen such a positive and hopeful evolution of treatment options for people with MS. I know I feel tremendously proud to be part of a specialist team where we've been able to shape patient care not only locally, but also on a national level.

I'm very firmly a 'nurse consultant,' not a 'consultant nurse' and I'm always very careful to make sure the word 'nurse' is the first thing that comes after my name. And we have a lot of different consultant positions in the United Kingdom in MS, so I'm not trying to make a criticism of anyone doing any role. But I whole-heartedly believe the sentiment of nurses remaining connected to their nursing roots is what will secure and sustain our specialty profession.

I've been in the right place at the right time for each of my career moves. Without a doubt I'm not the same person I was at the beginning of my career because I've had the opportunity to learn and be inspired by so many different people – both patients and colleagues – throughout the years. And I was also fortunate to realise the value in seizing any opportunity that came my way so as I could experience these different perspectives and triumphs.

If you want something enough, you'll look for a way to do it, even if it means a different way of achieving the end goal. And sometimes going about something in a different way gives you an alternate perspective that you can bring to the job. I may not have been trained to do what I'm doing in a traditional way or by taking a traditional path, but my combined experiences have given me what I need. And the same sentiment can be applied to people with MS. For any part of their life that might be taken away, I can guarantee they'll be able to find a way to achieve their goal, if they just think about it hard enough. It might not be conventional, and it might not be how they imagined, but I've heard time-after-time of people achieving what they need to through very imaginative means – and often doing it far better than they could have ever dreamed.

My hopes for the future treatment and management of MS:

• I have great hope that if we can identify the genetics that cause MS then we can tailor treatments to the individual. I'm excited about the prospect of personalised medicine.

• The explosion of treatment options has provided people with a greater choice to take a treatment that suits their lifestyle or addresses their symptoms.

• That the efficacy of the treatments will give people the courage to go out and have a normal life. In fact, I hope it empowers them to get on with life. Only two decades ago when you were diagnosed with MS, you were likely told to go home and rest. It's a very different conversation we have with the newly diagnosed now.

My advice for nurses beginning their career:

• Embrace every opportunity that comes your way.

• Don't stop asking questions.

• Never be afraid to say, 'I don't know.' MS is such a fast-changing specialty environment so if you stop asking questions, you're going to know less than you ever did and you will struggle.

• Learn from your patients and ask them things rather than just assuming. We use a technique called 'motivational interviewing' and I find it's helped our nurses look at things in a different way.

- And no matter what you're doing in the field, if there's something you're doing that you don't like, don't despair as you'll always take an experience away with you regardless.

- Use your national and international network to problem-solve and find out information.

- As a network we work hard and we play hard. I think sometimes as nurses we can forget we've got personal lives as well and it's really important to make sure you take care of yourself.

EDITH CINC
Melbourne, Australia

The nature of nursing is that you want to fix everything.
But the reality is you can't.

I've been a nurse since 1994. I did my training in the transition period in Australia where they took us from hospital-based programmes and into college training. In fact, the last lot of hospital trained nurses finished only six months before I started, so I began my career with the stigma of being one of 'those college-trained nurses.'

In the late 1970s, the Royal College of Nursing Australia pioneered a course that became the Diploma of Applied Science (Nursing), awarded by the Lincoln Institute in Melbourne and Cumberland College in Sydney. The transfer of nursing education to the university sector continued throughout the 1980s, and gradually hospital schools ceased operating. In the early 1990s, universities finally granted nursing education the same status as allied health and awarded bachelor's degrees in nursing rather than diplomas for entry-level courses.

The first move towards baccalaureate recognition was the

development of the Bachelor of Applied Science (Advanced Nursing), a post graduate degree that required registration as a registered nurse as a prerequisite to admission and completion of sixteen units. This course is no longer offered and has been superseded by the transition of 'post basic courses' conducted by various hospitals as a form of in-service training to the tertiary sector. The College of Nursing still runs post graduate certificate courses for nurses in many specialities.

The transfer of nursing education to the university sector from the hospital setting was the result of long-time efforts by leaders in Australian nursing. It was opposed by the medical hierarchy who viewed the development of highly trained professional nurses as a threat to their monopoly on the delivery of high-level health care. Many nurses themselves opposed the transfer on the grounds that hands-on experience in hospitals would be lost. One underlying cause of the opposition was that of societal views toward appropriate gender roles: Nursing as a 'female' profession and medicine as a 'male' profession.

It was quite interesting in those early years of the transition, having to do your graduate year and final training alongside the hospital-trained nurses who clearly demonstrated far superior clinical skills because of their hands-on experience. It was a difficult time. I can now see that nurses were trying to get some kind of academic recognition for their qualifications but the transitioning to achieve this was challenging and I didn't enjoy university; I felt at times the profession was being driven purely by the academia of the process rather than the practical side. I had to keep reminding myself of the reason why I wanted to become a nurse and put aside the feelings that the concept of hierarchy and sexism were at play and just remember that one day I wouldn't be the 'junior' of the profession. I had to believe that if I kept my head down and built up my expertise I'd eventually get to the point where I wasn't constantly looking over my shoulder to see what people were thinking.

I did my graduate year at the Royal Melbourne Hospital in Australia with a placement on the renal ward – an environment that provided me a good deal of hands-on experience for my foundational skills. After graduation, I travelled overseas for a few months and when I returned to the Royal Melbourne I went into a pool of nurses. This pool meant that I was assigned to cover a variety of wards. It was quite interesting to discover that the wards and specialities I thought I'd enjoy, I didn't, and vice versa. One assignment was to a bone marrow transplant ward. At that stage I didn't even fully understand what a bone marrow transplant was, let alone how to look after the patients! But curiously, I kept being re-assigned to this ward and came to find a bizarre affinity with the work. It was very intensive nursing behind closed doors but the team were absolutely incredible; so supportive and wonderful. Nurses for roles in that particular area of the oncology wing were in high demand, but having lost my father to cancer, I never thought I'd be inclined to work in such an environment. Low and behold I was offered a permanent role in the bone marrow transplant unit and ended up becoming a clinical nurse specialist in haematology, oncology, and bone marrow transplant and that eventually sealed my introduction to the early stem cell transplant trials in multiple sclerosis back in the 1990s.

At that stage I'd looked after a few people with MS and also worked on clinical trials for haematology and oncology. I was always a clinical nurse and never wanted to go into management roles but my desire to learn was always so strong and I was fortunate to have great mentors and educators.

I had been practising nursing for about ten years – primarily in those clinical areas – when I had my first child. On my return from maternity leave I discovered I really wanted to work a bit closer to home. I had recently met a nurse at a conference overseas who was the Clinical Research Associate (CRA) for a pharma-ceutical company. Whilst the role of the CRA's is a little different these days, back then her job was to help sites coordinate clinical trials using the treatments her company was developing. She was basically the go-between for the hospital and clinical staff and the pharmaceutical company in answering any questions and ensuring adherence to ethical conduct and trial processes for the clinical trial of treatments.

Belinda – the CRA – and I ended up getting to know each other very well and she was now working at Austin Health managing the Cancer Trials Centre. Quite serendipitously, the Austin was closer to home, I'd worked extensively in oncology trials and was friendly with Belinda; a transfer to the Austin was a natural move for me.

My life in MS is really a product of circumstance and after about 18 months of working in the oncology trials at Austin, Belinda mentioned a new MS drug that was ready to be trialled. It coincided with a personal desire to move into a different area. The drug being trialled was a monoclonal antibody called Lemtrada (Alemtuzumab). The Austin Hospital was looking for someone to run the studies and they were having difficulty finding people with enough expertise. At this stage, the other monoclonal antibody (Tysabri) wasn't even available in Australia, so there just weren't many nurses who'd had much experience in the field. My background working in haematology had given me that experience and once again, the move seemed like an obvious one. It was a new challenge, because whilst I knew quite a bit about managing a clinical trial, I knew very little about multiple sclerosis. Serendipitously, there were actually two positions available for the Lemtrada trial and both Belinda and I ended up becoming a team!

At this point, the only knowledge I had of MS were the three or so patients I'd seen in the oncology ward who were receiving their treatments there. I clearly remember my new boss in the Lemtrada trial saying to me "you do realise that MS is a pretty common disease, don't you?" because I really didn't have that perspective. I didn't personally know anyone with MS so its prevalence didn't fully register at the time.

Isn't it funny that once you start working in MS or meet one person with MS, then you start recognising exactly how prevalent it is! I came to find out I actually knew plenty of people with MS but I had never realised they were living with it. To be honest, it was a completely eye-opening experience.

***

There is no 'one size fits all' approach...

My days in oncology provided me a great deal of experience to be able to work alongside people living with MS. They are two entirely different diseases, but I've been able to draw some parallels that can benefit my patients. I know I can never be completely in the shoes of someone living with MS – and ideally the disease wouldn't even exist – but I'm intent on helping them through their journey and a decade in oncology has given me a unique perspective. I think when people can look at other disease courses and the treatments that have been developed for those conditions, it does provide a wider perspective and certainly hope.

When my patients find out I went from oncology to MS they joke that I've gone from one morbid disease to another, but I always resolutely explain to them that people can live extremely well with MS.

And as strange as it sounds, I feel like I've come into MS at a really great time. Never has there been so many treatment choices for people and it's exciting to see the transition of therapies from research to approval. It's actually mind blowing! When I explain to newly diagnosed patients that only ten years ago we didn't have the type of drugs in Australia that we do now and exactly how much more effective they are, they're always amazed.

One of the things I found quite interesting from the onset of my career in MS was the difference in how the doctors dealt with new treatments. The oncologists seemed far less risk-adverse than the neurologists when it came to new therapies. I've been at the forefront of the introduction of Lemtrada and Tysabri in Australia and have seen how hopeful the neurologists are with these treatments but also how cautious they are with these newer and more powerful disease modifying therapies (DMTs). It's a good thing and the reality is that we know far less about multiple sclerosis than cancer.

Of course, the other glaring difference between the treatment of cancer and the treatment of MS is that there is no 'one size fits all' approach. In cancer treatments, we have more structure and time-proven ways to treat the various cancers. The protocols of cancer treatments are fairly regimented and the side effects or outcomes are somewhat more predictable. MS throws up so many variables, and the symptoms are so unique amongst people and that induces a lot of confusion and fear. In cancer, we generally know how people will react to treatments, what their recovery will involve and I guess the various timeframes of everything. But with MS, there may be no end date to the fatigue or pain or impairment and this can cause a lot of anxiety for people. Dealing with fear of the unknown is very destabilising.

In my experience, cancer is very different to MS when we look at the impact of disclosure as well. Cancer comes in and generally has a very immediate and devastating effect and it's quite difficult not to disclose that you have cancer. But with MS, we describe it as an invisible disease because its symptoms (and treatments) are not always so obvious. But this invisibility can also make it harder for someone to come to terms with a diagnosis of MS. With cancer, there's less possibility to do that. Cancer's sense of urgency, in having to have surgery and undergo rigorous treatments, such as chemotherapy and radiotherapy, has a massive and immediate impact on your life. Whereas MS is about putting the brakes on and slowing down. For us as nurses, helping patients understand what they're dealing with and making sure they understand their disease is quite individual and so are the treatments options... And it can take time to unravel all of that.

Destigmatising the perception of what MS is like to live with is a big part of my job, not only amongst my patients, but publically as well. Some of the tools I use to displace the stigma are talking about the inspiring people I've met who live with MS but also, at a base level, just explaining that because MS can be quite invisible, it's likely that everyone knows someone with MS but they never realised it.

That individuality of MS presents some interesting challenges at times. For me, the mental health issues have been some of the hardest to navigate. Obviously, you develop some counselling skills from your nursing training, but I've had some very confronting situations over the years, particularly when it comes to a patient's personal safety in times of poor mental health.

And just not being able to help a patient enough – in the way you'd really like to – can be frustrating. I wish I could do more but, in some situations, I feel I'm limited in skills, or time or resources or even the physical ability to do more.

More recently, dealing with the administration of the various government agencies and programmes that are designed to assist patients has also become a mine field for me. I almost feel like every person with MS needs a personal case manager just to help them phone or communicate with these agencies, along with keeping up to date on the various intricacies of their programmes. Not long ago I'd just say 'yeah, send me your forms and I'll fill everything out for you,' but I know that's not sustainable, so now I'm developing strategies to expedite and streamline the process for everyone – the patients, their families, the nurses and even the doctors. It's through no fault of anyone in particular, but modernising medicine and health care means that many of the services and resources that once existed are now obsolete, disbanded or unobtainable and keeping up with that changing landscape is frustrating.

The nature of nursing is that you want to fix everything. But the reality is you can't.

***

I ultimately aim to empower my patients to take control over this thing...

I've been working in MS for a decade and I know now the first thing I need to do with a newly diagnosed patient is tap into their psyche. I try to do this from the onset, despite the fact that we know they're bewildered about so many things right after being told "you have MS." But in those ensuing consultations, a lot of what I talk about with my patients is to get them to just put the brakes on; to explain that taking a little time to process and adjust is okay; that we're here to help on this journey; that there's no urgency.

I talk about what MS actually is – in layman's terms – and the simple pathology of the disease; but I also find it important to start introducing the notion that medicine offers one aspect of treatment but additionally, there is a myriad of ways they can help themselves. I ultimately aim to empower my patients to take control over this thing. Hopefully they see that there's so many ways they can have input into their own disease course. I can't stress how important it is for people living with MS to understand that medicines are only one of the aspects of managing the disease – that the lifestyle factors are also key – and that not everything needs to be addressed all at once.

Understandably those first few months are critical in assessing someone's support network, personal mindset and resilience. If I can work out whether they're likely to start isolating themselves, have tendencies towards depression or anxiety or simply don't have a healthy, strong or rational support network, then I can identify those who are potentially the most vulnerable.

For the person living with MS it's really important to have someone solid on your team and it's not always the obvious person. It may not be the spouse or parent of a patient. It might be an aunt with a medical background who is a far better advocate for the patient, because they leave any hysteria or irresponsibility out of the process.

My primary message is that I am here to help you continue to live the life you want to live, and I am here to support and guide you in those goals.

***

Everyone is different, but we'll piece the jigsaw puzzle together.

I find the newly diagnosed need the support and resources of MS nurses much more in that early phase. I constantly re-assure my patients that it's okay to ask questions and seek reassurance and that all these questions are helping them to develop skills and knowledge to take better control of the MS. In time they will need us less as they learn more about their own disease course; and we're there to travel that disease course with them.

The first thing I say to a person newly diagnosed with MS is "you will be okay." And there's an artform to saying that simple line convincingly but with empathy and authority. I then reassure that I'm there to help them better understand what is happening to their body and help them on this journey for as long as it takes. Initially I'd love for my patients to understand that in time they will be able to look back and know that they aren't going to be as scared, and that they are okay.

Early on, I really want my patients to understand the concept that they can take control in looking after themselves in so many ways – mentally, emotionally and physically. Perhaps they could consider taking the focus off the disease specifically, and to instead look at their body as a whole.

Naturally I get asked about diet and nutrition a lot. People want to know if there's a specific diet or something in particular they should or shouldn't eat. I'll only talk about diet and nutrition in a generic fashion. I think the patient making up their own mind about diet gives them a sense of control. We don't have a lot of control over the disease in general terms but patients can take control over what they eat and how to look after themselves. And I think embracing those habits early empowers the patient to look after themselves at any point of their disease course.

And encouraging social engagement is also really important. I want my patients to enjoy their life and feel fulfilled, be it via friendships or experiences or contribution through work or community.

Another thing I find really valuable is urging my patients to grant themselves some time and space. It's okay to just stop for a second, pull back and allow themselves to be objective and measured about stuff. Often my opening question in a consultation is 'what's your biggest concern today?' And it should go without saying that time to grieve in those early days – crying and letting emotion out – is also an important part of the process. And if someone with MS can't do it in my office then where can they do it? Giving people the permission to be vulnerable with you also builds rapport.

Honesty is so important to me and I don't mince my words. I'll explain that the therapies aren't perfect; they're 'disease modifying.' I'll use statistics to illustrate a point but also be careful to clarify that "statistics don't apply to individuals." It's one of my favourite lines. When you've worked in clinical research, as I have, and then comparing therapies for patients, you realise that the statistics and measurements mean very different things to different people. A scientist on a clinical trial for a DMT is obviously going to be looking at relapse rates as a standard measurement. And this statistic then becomes part of the literature that the patient reads. But it is not an individual indication. These statistics are averaged and again – very important information for a researcher but not particularly relevant to an individual. Some people get far better results and unfortunately some people get a worse result, but we're so much more advanced than we were a decade ago and have multiple options to find the best fit for each patient. I can't stress enough to the patients that everyone is different, and we'll piece the jigsaw puzzle together. And to that end, getting upset from the things you hear relating to other people, on other therapies, is not helpful or constructive.

The other primary thing I tell patients is to put aside the historical data about treatments. The patients diagnosed today are going to have a very different future than the patients diagnosed twenty years ago. And that is due to the advent of new therapies and better MRI techniques and our understanding of how to treat active disease.

And the notion of disclosure in MS also works in another way. I need my patients to feel like they can disclose things to me so as I can help them. I see all too commonly in those early days that friends and family will Google information or buy books or make treatment suggestions to the person living with MS. It's their way of offering support and trying to find a connection in the MS journey. But there's a time and place for all of this information and I spend a lot of time in those early days of diagnosis unwinding some of the anxiety or outright inaccuracies of this 'helpful' information which has been offered.

Some of the first questions a newly diagnosed patient will most commonly ask is if they will need to stop work, will they need to sell their house and move? Will their children get MS? And these are all scary things for a person to contemplate because they're a large part of someone's life. As time goes on, most of the questions tend to revolve around new treatment options – particularly as more choices are becoming available – and then of course the risk versus benefit of those various treatments compared to what they're currently on. For some patients, they choose not to take a DMT from the beginning but they still keep in touch and keep coming back to me year after year. I think there's a feeling of safety and connection for them in that.

I'd like to think I've got it all figured out but people continue to surprise me every single day.

The inspiring patients to me are the ones who absolutely make the best of what they have. It might be a patient who is living with secondary progressive MS but they still do their gym work every day. They are hell bent on maximising everything they are still able to do, rather than things they cannot.

And those that are focussed on exercise and actively helping themselves are in a much better frame of mind and mentally stronger to take anything on. Anecdotally I can definitely see the correlation between people who choose to help themselves, are the ones who are better able to control the disease. And to be honest, it's those people who make our jobs easier because they are such great ambassadors to other patients to live better lives with MS.

Understandably, it's very difficult for most people at the time of diagnosis to be able to look forward. But I continue to impress upon the newly diagnosed that they might not remember much detail of what I say in those early conversations but they need to remember and recognise that they will look back on things and think 'Yep, okay... None of that was too bad.' It takes a year or so but that deep seated panic does subside. They will get through this stuff and some people even tell me what a blessing the diagnosis has been. And let's face it.... whether we like it or not, life has to go on and does go on.

***

We all have bad days and also those times where twenty percent of my patients will take up eighty percent of my time. But I don't really have the time to dwell on the bad days. I'm extremely lucky I have an exceptional team of nurses I work with; we're lucky to have each other and a strong enough relationship to just say what we think. And there is therapy in that – in being able to release a bit of our frustration and emotion amongst ourselves; amongst colleagues who just 'get it.'

The relationship with my colleagues is so very important and because we all practice similarly and I admire them as nurses, we're all on the same page in how to deal with things. And we can just be ourselves and that in itself is a huge advantage. As much as we're here to give support to others, I'm grateful to have the support of my colleagues to support me too. I often wonder about other nurses who work in isolation and think it must be really difficult for them. I don't know if I could do it; but as nurses, we do what we have to do to get ourselves through the situation. And let's face it, often we're so busy that the only option is to just get through things. I could have a hideous consultation where I'm banging my head against a brick wall and just not getting through to the patient – for a multitude of reasons – and then have to back it up with the next consultation, which might be a patient who's a refugee. And those consultations are so much more complex.

In fact, it's really confronting dealing with a lot of new things that we've never had to deal with in the past. Situations like the refugee population we're looking after in Melbourne. MS can be the least of their issues if they've come from a war-torn country. They have a different context on problems and in turn, it gives us a different angle on life's issues. It can put parts of life into perspective when you're working with vulnerable patients such as those from the refugee network. These patients often have complex and chronic physical and mental health conditions – some of which have been unrecognised for far too long and others that are newly developed because of the conditions they've escaped from. I have patients who are more worried about the nightmares their children are having or the bombings in the places they've run from, and I have to then tell them that they also have MS. Most are non-English speaking and so terrified and scared. It blows my mind and it's tremendously confronting at times.

Fridays are our primary clinic day and that afternoon, we all convene for a round table discussion to recap every patient from the day's clinic, along with other patients from the week that require further debriefing. Generally, there's about eight of us, including the neurologists who work in the MS clinic, their fellows and the registrars, along with the three nurses from our neuro-immunology team. These round tables are obviously valuable from a patient management perspective but also tremendously important as a way of supporting each other. We all learn from and contribute to each other's cases and it also goes a long way in feeling like part of the team. I love that it's a time that we get to ask some pretty detailed questions of our Director of Neurology and problem solve issues with him. First and foremost, it benefits our patients but it serves to strengthen our nursing expertise. It's very much a holistic approach and there's great power in pooling that knowledge.

Have I ever had a situation I didn't know how to fix? Yes....many! And if I really sat back and tried to determine the common thread to these challenges, I'd have to conclude that they come from those situations where the dynamic of the consultation is just incredibly confrontational or fuelled with tension. In these situations, it won't be an actual physical or medical thing I can't fix. It's about the mindset of the patient or a tension in the relationship we have together, which could be present for a number of reasons. If I sense a challenge like this emerging, I'll nearly always get a colleague to take the patient consultation. It's important to me that our patients get the best care possible and if I'm unsure if I can remain objective, I will want the patient to speak with someone else.

I've learned over the years there may be times I need to step back and admit that the patient would be better served by a colleague than myself. And I know my colleagues in the clinic go through the exact same experience and that we can all support each other in this. It's a matter of recognising each other's skills and limitations. And I also recognise it's an absolute luxury to be able to share the load with my team mates. In my clinic, I'm known as the nurse who best handles the patients who are upset and crying. Another nurse is really great at working with the angry and aggressive consults. We all juggle according to our strengths.

Most of the time I think I'm pretty good at pacifying a situation. I'm deeply empathetic and I also believe you have to allow people just to 'be.' You have to give them space to go through the emotions in their own timeframes and also work out things for themselves.

My role is to interject into this process with the patient and work out where we can help.

As nurses, we're trained not to give advice, but more to assist the patients in navigating whatever they're going through. It's really interesting but also increasingly difficult with more therapies becoming available each year. Some patients really struggle with the process of not being definitively told what type of therapy to go on. For one, it can make the consultations a lot longer. I could easily spend up to two hours with a newly diagnosed person working through the process of explaining a variety of DMTs. And then I could repeat it all the next week with the same patient when they've had time to process and figure out the questions they want to ask. And believe me for every question asked and answered, you then create a myriad of peripheral questions. It could be anything from other medical conditions or side-effects right through to something they saw on a current affairs programme two months ago. For us, we have to ensure we're all over the media coverage of people with MS or new treatments or whatever over-dramatised thing they might be broadcasting that week.

You can always tell when the media have said something about MS because our phones ring more often than usual. We even get calls from interstate – often angry calls – because the caller may have heard we're offering a treatment or a trial that they don't have access to in their state. Or a family member of a patient will call and quiz us as to why we can't give their loved one a particular therapy; it's potentially awkward. But I have to be both kind and firm to guard our resources and also our medical responsibility and liability. I hate these conversations. I hate taking away hope.

The litigious nature of society has changed the way I talk to patients. I'll often repeat warnings to the same person in every consultation no matter how many times they've seen me or how sensible I believe them to be. It's just not worth taking the risk that a patient may be having a bad cognitive day or simply misinterpreting things. It could be something as simple as a reminder about shortened operating hours over Christmas right through to medication protocols. And I don't care how often the patient tells me that I've already told them! We'll make a joke out of it, but I find myself being very careful to cover every base; it protects the patient as much as myself.

On the flip side, I'll have patients who incessantly call and ask the same question because they're waiting to hear the answer they want to hear. But I can't always give the answer they want. And it's frustrating that I can't give them what they want, and it would be even more frustrating for my patient. Often there's more than MS going on for the patient. For me, if I identify this pattern where a patient repeatedly asks the same question, I'll start working out whether the situation is masking something deeper going on – either mentally or emotionally – or whether the question isn't being answered the way the patient wants because they actually want to ask something entirely different to what they're saying. It's part mind reading, part reading between the lines and all the while making sure you're not giving unwarranted advice. I've had many, many conversations where we just go around in circles.

In the instances where I identify that a patient may need to seek support from a mental health professional, it's then a fine line in diplomatically suggesting that the patient speak with a psychologist and the patient taking offence because they think you're suggesting they have mental problems. It's really difficult. And you don't want to destroy your interpersonal relationship with the patient, but you want to make sure they're getting the best help from the most appropriate person.

As nurses, I think it would be inherent in most of us to want to help as much as possible. And part of that is wanting to offer advice.

So I think a good skill to learn is how to deliver advice without offering it.

For example, someone with a history of an eating disorder or the underlying psychological traits of an eating disorder will not want to take a steroid treatment and will query the neurologist's prescription or simply not comply with the treatment, no matter how much we know it will help the patient's relapses. My conversation with a patient like this will set out all the facts about their disease course with MS, summarise our previous conversations and the treatment decisions and then recount the patient's own queries about the treatment. I'll bring it full circle by asking them what it is they'd like to achieve and what help they'd like from our clinic? I'll also remind them that sometimes, as a patient, it can be difficult to remain objective and that there are times that you need to surrender yourself to the health professionals and allow them to care for you in the way they know best. Sometimes it's as outright as asking 'what do you think might happen to you if you don't take this treatment for three days?' As nurses, we have to figure out (and generally pretty quickly) what it is that's holding them back from complying with the best medical treatment for them.

Each consultation has to be tailored to the patient's psyche and individual concerns. And that's where building the rapport with each person is so important. But also the realisation that there are limitations in what we can do. If a person isn't being compliant with their appointments, we can't set out to do everything for them – like pay for their parking or search for a dog sitter... but we can aim to remove the excuses that aren't really stacking up.

I'm passionate about clinical nursing: I'm good at general patient care and I want to do that for as long as possible. I'm trained to be a nurse, not an administrator. I'm trained to assess a patient's needs and my role in the health care system is to fulfil that as best I can. And it's my fellow clinical team members who allow me to do all of that to the high standard I set for myself. I feel very lucky I have the luxury of time to spend with my patients and it's an absolute investment in their empowerment to manage the disease and live the best life they can.

Quite simply, you know you are making a difference. That is why we do what we do.

My hopes for the future treatment and management of MS:

- I often think about where the great hope for MS treatments will come from. There is obviously plenty of talk about stem cells, and the knowledge I've gained from my previous life as a nurse in bone marrow transplants has been helpful in understanding the ramifications of AHSCT for multiple sclerosis.

- The development of remyelinating agents would be incredible for people living with MS.

- I also aspire for us to figure out how to put a halt to the disease without the nasty side effects.

- I'm really interested to see advancements in MRI techniques and mapping and understanding brain volume. Having the ability to map brain volume over time might be a way to better develop drug treatments.

- My other hope for how we treat the disease is by means of scientist retention in Australia and around the world; that we actually have the money to enable greater and ongoing research and the scientists could dedicate more time to science and less time to applying for grants. I think the incredible minds of the world are grossly under-valued. In the corporate world, people with this level of intelligence would be paid a fortune, but in the scientific world they struggle from grant to grant. The pursuit of science is so admirable to me.

My advice for nurses beginning their career:

•   Utilise the expertise around you, be it from your own workplace or through the specialist nursing groups. I've been lucky enough to work alongside some of the best MS nurses in this country and they continue to inspire as much as educate us to be the best clinical nurses we can.

•   We are so lucky in our profession that we can make a difference to the lives of others. We're not well paid but our jobs are incredibly satisfying because for the large majority of patients, we do make a huge difference. It always outweighs the situations where you can't help.

•   Remember that the frustrations of the role are far outweighed by the positive outcomes we see every day.

•   Implore your patients to avoid randomly Googling things which are concerning them and instead direct them to the appropriate sites.

ANNE KRAKAU HANSEN
Copenhagen, Denmark

Be the master of MS; do not let it become the master of you.

....

I began my first years of nursing in Denmark in 1983. For the first seven years of my career, I tried different rotations amongst the fields of general medical, rheumatological, surgical and even psychiatry at the Slagelse Sygehus Hospital in the southern Danish region of Zealand. I found my way into neurological nursing in 1990, enjoying it so much that I became a specialist MS nurse in 1996 and only a decade later, was promoted to become the head nurse of the Danish Multiple Sclerosis Centre in Copenhagen.

The Danish Multiple Sclerosis Center (DMSC) comprises the MS Clinics at Rigshospitalet Glostrup and Rigshospitalet Blegdamsvej, the Optic Neuritis Clinic at Rigshospitalet Glostrup, the MS Re-search Units at both locations, and the Neuroimmunology Laboratory at Rigshospitalet Blegdamsvej. The centre is the largest MS clinic in Denmark and altogether, we have sixteen nurses who specialise in assisting MS patients with the service being funded by our national taxation system.

I am one of the longest serving nurses in Denmark in the field of MS and I was actually head-hunted into the DMSC in 1996 because of my experience in neurological nursing. It was at a time that we were starting to experience the introduction of the disease modifying therapies (DMTs) into the country and specialists were required to monitor the treatments and help the patients.

In Denmark, there are approximately 17,000 people living with multiple sclerosis – the third highest-rate per capita in the world behind just San Marino and Canada. Denmark has a population of some 5.77 million people. Right now, according to Finn Sellebjerg, a doctor at the Sclerosis Centre and the Rigshospitalet city hospital, there is nothing obvious to explain why Denmark has such a high rate of the illness.

In my outpatient clinic, we support around 4,000 patients in total and as the lead nurse at the clinic, I could see up to 80 patients in a day. I like to at least touch base with as many people as possible and then also provide support to the other nurses in their consultations or DMT infusions. Understandably, my days are quite full!

Some of the most challenging situations I face as a MS nurse are providing care for paediatric and adolescent patients. We see some of the youngest patients in the country at my clinic. In those early days of treating the children, I found it quite hard emotionally. Our youngest patients were around twelve years old and we had about twenty registered with our clinic.

Understandably it can be so difficult to talk to children about a disease such as MS whilst also trying to educate them. I found that they simply wanted to be doing other things in life, the same as their friends were; they certainly don't want to be sick and undergoing treatments. But now we have many more services, such paediatric neurologists and psychologists and we've also trained MS nurses specifically for this area.

***

It's actually quite wonderful to see how people adapt.

In those early days of being diagnosed, most patients tend to want to know about treatments and how to care for themselves with MS, but as the fog of the news of the diagnosis starts to lift, they also want to know 'what next?' and 'what will happen to me?'

And as nurses, we can't always give them the answers to these questions other than to encourage patients to live positively and know that life can still be quite good. And that's not to say that we underestimate how difficult it is to live with MS, but I believe instilling a positive mindset from the start is just so beneficial. I still think it takes a year or two for people living with MS to fully understand and reconcile the diagnosis and everything that comes with it and then they can see that life does go on.

Perhaps it takes a bit of practice and experimentation to craft the coping techniques and strong mentality to live well with MS. And I can see it takes time and the experience of talking to friends and family and even other people living with MS for a newly diagnosed person to grasp that they have a support network. I think it's at this point – when they realise they have formed their own little support group – that they feel confident knowing that moving forward in life is not only possible but could be even better than before. Once the newly diagnosed start seeing that what they are going through is also experienced and felt by others, then they start to feel normal, or at least a new sense of normal.

As the years go by, I see many patients re-considering what is important to them in their life and certainly re-prioritising what it is they want to achieve. It's actually quite wonderful to see how people adapt.

A big part of our role as MS nurses is guiding people to get through various life challenges and decisions. We do find ourselves being counsellors at times; we deal with so much more than just medications and physical concerns. And throughout my thirty-year career as a MS nurse, much of my training in this particular area has been 'on the job.'

I know our patients feel a great degree of relief that they have a dedicated clinic such as ours; a place that they can rely on to understand what they are dealing with and where they don't have to re-explain everything from the start each time. Having to constantly explain a health history can be quite exhausting. And always talking about acute health situations can be stressful for people as well. But we must always remember that as much as we're training on the job to care for our patients, so too are those people living with MS 'training on the job' to learn about the disease and how to best care for themselves.

When I first started out, I had MS patients that I really couldn't do much for. They would come to us, get diagnosed and we would then send them home with the advice to stay strong and be positive. But now, we know so much more. We have a lot more options to be able to provide for our patients and be can aim for better outcomes.

We have some fifteen-plus DMT's available in Denmark, which is certainly in line with what's available around the world. This is fantastic news for our patients because the choice of medication is an important decision. However, it's also an enormous undertaking for our MS nurses in Denmark to ensure they are comprehensively educated in each of the DMTs and also remain up-to-date in their training of the monitoring and administration of each drug. I see this factor becoming a huge burden in our profession. We are similar to many other countries where the neurologist will be the primary health care professional to suggest the best DMT to fit the patient's own situation, but as nurses, we're probably more relied upon to monitor the patient as they take their treatments and ensure it remains a good fit, not just clinically but also that the DMT fits their lifestyle.

There is a very good system of care in Denmark for people living with MS and my advice to those newly diagnosed can be quite simple at times: We now know so much more than we ever did about how to treat the disease but also, to embrace good lifestyle choices as those simple adjustments alone can make living with MS far healthier and more comfortable. I try to point out examples of how so many people around the world are living remarkably well with MS.

But one of the biggest things I like to impress upon the newly diagnosed is that you have to be the 'master of MS; do not let it become the master of you.' I like my patients to know that as MS nurses we are always there to help and guide, but they really have to learn how to handle their own lives and take control as much as possible.

And that's probably why some of the most uplifting things I see at work are also the simplest. It's when a patient might visit the clinic with her newborn baby, and I realise that she's had the courage to overcome any fears and get on with life and build a family. Or those patients who find a way to keep on doing the things that bring them joy or build their life, such as running a marathon or continuing their education. These are the people who are the master of their MS!

***

TAKING CONTROL COMPASSIONATELY

It's not always easy to make the time to look after yourself in the roles we play, but somehow we all seem to get through! At the clinic, we make an effort to regularly check in with each other and also at our nursing conferences, we discuss how to help and support one-another more effectively. As our clinic's leader, I also ensure that our nurses attend symposia and work-shops that keep them up-to-date with time management techniques and also undertake personal health and wellness programmes.

But I just believe it's an inherent character we possess as both women and professional carers to want to keep looking after others all the time. For nearly all of us at the clinic – and I imagine many other hospitals around the world – we do what we love in caring for others all day and then we go home and care for our families and children at night because again, we love it. It's not a conscious thought process; we just do it! But all the same, finding some type of balance is terribly important so as we have the time and energy to do the things we love. My experience has shown me that being comfortable in your workplace and surrounding yourself with a good team is very important, as is ensuring that everyone on your team understands each other.

One of the greatest challenges I've faced over the course of my career is working out how to deal with the increasing volume of patients. The increased workload and strain on resources became very evident to me when I was promoted to the leadership role at my clinic.

With the promotion came the responsibility of talking with the clinic directors about how we could manage these problems. One of the things I advocated for at the clinic was to foster strong time management skills amongst my entire team whilst at the same time, ensuring we taught our patients that there was also a limit to the type of things we could do for them. I think it's okay to coach your patients that there's certain tasks their general practitioner may be better suited to assist with.

It can be really difficult to always be realistic about how much time or energy we actually have to do things for our patients; we need to learn to spread the workload a bit, but we're not very good at doing this! I think the earlier we inspire and empower the patients to be a major part of managing their own health care, the better. Like I said before – and this goes for both the patients and MS nurses – become the master of MS; do not let it become the master of you.

My thirty-year career has seen a tremendous amount of change in how we 'master' MS. In the 1990s when I first started my career as a neurological nurse, there were no DMTs for the treatment of multiple sclerosis. And then only six years into my career we had two treatments; fast forward to some three decades later and we have over fifteen DMTs. My personal journey has been one of working with just a few treatments in a small clinic to now managing many, many treatments is the country's largest clinic.

During this time, it's been exciting for me to see the global collaboration in how we manage MS go from strength-to-strength.

My hopes for the future treatment and management of MS:

- Obviously, we want to be able to find a cure for MS, but I think it would be both tremendously helpful – not to mention fascinating – to understand how MS develops in the first place.

- My hope is that we can drive many more dollars into research to understand the cause and then develop a cure. At the moment I see the area of treatments being funded more-so than the pursuit of finding the cause or a cure.

My advice for nurses beginning their career:

- First and foremost, listen to the patient! Listen intently to what they're telling you and what they feel, as you'll learn a lot. This is especially important when we have to rely on the patient's first-hand account of what they're experiencing so we can effectively manage their symptoms.

- I think our culture in Denmark makes for patients who are very open and direct, and this helps us enormously. But when we do work with patients who are a little more reserved or shy to talk about certain aspects of MS, we can help them open up by sharing stories about how other patients might deal with things.

- Of course, every patient is different and I think it's a great skill for us to develop as nurses in being able to read individuals and work out how to make them comfortable.

ADRIANA CARTWRIGHT
Victoria, Australia

Often my role isn't fixing the problem but at least getting the patient on a path towards a solution.

A s a high school student, I was always intrigued by the jobs where I could help people. Those jobs like nursing or emergency services or going into the fire brigade or police force. Basically, I wanted to be of service and do something that had a practical component. I could never see myself sitting in an administrative role. First and foremost, it was the practical side of any role that would appeal to me; I loved helping people and I've always found myself thriving in a team environment.

Maybe it's because both my husband and I are one of six children and then we also have three teenage children ourselves, so we're never short of people and family and commitments. But I've never really thought about the reason I wanted to pursue roles where I could be of service. It's just something deeply ingrained in me.

When I was working towards for my Bachelor of Nursing in the early '90s, we were able to pick any topic – any condition at all – as part of an in-depth research assignment, and out of the thousands of things I could have chosen, I chose multiple sclerosis. Looking back, I often think 'what made me pick MS?' And I don't really know; I think it was because I loved neurology and have always loved studying the brain and wondering how it works. And of course, I've always loved interacting with people and found a fascination with the psychology of social interactions. And then again, maybe the fact that MS is a young person's illness affecting mostly women resonated more emotionally with me; or perhaps I saw the advertisements for the MS Read-a-thon on television (complete with people sitting in wheelchairs). Curiously, I hadn't known anyone diagnosed with MS at that point, so I'm not a hundred percent sure why I chose MS as my topic, but I was just drawn to studying the condition even back then. Can you believe I've actually kept that presentation from university as well!!

And whilst I may have chosen MS as my specialty study, it was only after seventeen years of working on the neurology wards that I eventually found myself quite serendipitously becoming a dedicated MS nurse.

On obtaining my Bachelor of Nursing in 1994, I began working at St Vincent's Hospital in Melbourne as a registered nurse. The next year I was able to concentrate on my love of neurosciences in both the neurology and neurosurgery departments as a Clinical Nurse Specialist and later as an Associate Nurse Unit Manager. I was just so passionate about the work I was doing and wanted to cement the knowledge with a diploma in Frontline Management and eventually a post-graduate certificate in neurosciences nursing.

After spending about a decade in these roles, I followed a new challenge in becoming the clinical nurse educator for the post-graduate neurosciences course. This then led to a project in stroke education and the coordination of an integrated stroke prevention clinical trial within the neurosciences department at St Vincent's.

Once the trial finished up, I was asked to do a small stint covering for a MS nurse on long-service leave; she subsequently moved to a new hospital after her leave and I can happily say I've been absorbed in the world of MS since!

My on-the-job training for MS may have been a bit different to most because I fell into this role. In fact, for the first few months I felt as if the patients all knew more than I did. It was a truly awful feeling. There were times I'd have to rely on the doctors quite a lot and I could sometimes feel myself back-peddling. But all those feelings made me examine what I was doing and simply more determined to learn from the situations; and with time, you can't help but to become better – and more intuitive – about things.

I'm really fortunate that I've been in the neurology wards of St Vincent's Hospital for over twenty-two years and this has allowed me to forge strong relationships with the neurologists and doctors I work with. When you're dealing with a disease like MS where there's so many variables – in symptoms, treatments and disease progress – it's great to have that stabilising factor of knowing so well the team you work with. We all know a lot about the same things in different ways and it's good to come together to work out the solution.

***

The treatment of MS has certainly come a long way since my university days. Back then we only had a few injectables such as Copaxone and interferons to treat patients. I remember a workshop very early in my nursing career where a MS nurse demonstrated how to draw up an interferon treatment and then inject it into the patient and that was the first time we were seeing drugs like this.

Generally, when I first see my newly diagnosed patients, I find they hold their emotions together quite well, at least while they're with the neurologists. Perhaps because the neurology consults can feel a bit more clinical and the patients strive to keep a stiff upper lip.

But I can sense the shift in mood prior to our appointment together. No doubt there's something about anticipating the appointment day, combined with the sombre wait in the clinic's reception room. I'll greet my new patients and then lead them down to my office and at that point, they just burst into tears. A sense of expectation and mounting fear has undoubtedly built and this is the time when the patients just let it all out. The doctors joke with me that I must have shares in Kleenex!

In that first appointment, I'll often start with a simple question such as:

- 'How was your appointment with the neurologist?'
- Or 'what's your understanding of everything so far?'

I find questions like that can bring me up to speed very quickly on the patient's understanding of what their neurologist may have said, the level of comprehension as to what is going on and where the patient is at, regardless of what the medical records in front of me say. It can help cut through any issues of miscommunication or misunderstanding very quickly.

But truthfully, in that first meeting there's not a lot of pressure to ask too many questions but instead I simply sit with them and let them feel the emotion of what's going on. I'll allow them to direct the conversation to what they need it to achieve at that point in time.

I'll just reassure my patients and let them know there's treatment options and that we work together with the neurologist to find something to suit them. Often the neurologist will have already discussed therapies with them but at this point in their diagnosis there's so much information and a great deal just goes in one ear and out the other.

And sometimes there's still uncertainty about the diagnosis in general. It could be that the patient is still trying to process things, or perhaps they're just optimistic people who believe that the exacerbation was a one-off event and will never happen again.

Most importantly, I don't want to overwhelm anyone in those first consultations.

And whilst everyone is different, in that immediate time after diagnosis, there's not really a heap of questions that the patients will think to ask. I find it's often not until after the patient and their family have gone home and had a day or even a week to process everything and then they'll start ruminating over the various aspects of the diagnosis. It's then that the questions will come! And those questions will certainly vary depending on a person's age, level of education, lifestyle and where they're at in life. I also find that how a person deals with MS can be influenced by whether they personally know someone else living with the disease. The direct association with MS will shape their impressions and provide the picture for them. To be honest, when a newly diagnosed patient knows someone with MS, I find they're actually a bit more optimistic and realistic.

But there are definitely exceptions to this rule, and it tends to be in patients who are diagnosed later in life. One of the trickiest things I'll need to overcome with them is that they're not going to automatically end up in a wheelchair. This cohort have all grown up in a time when the ads for MS fundraising relied heavily on imagery of wheelchair-bound people; the 'wheelchair question' is the first thing they'll ask me and in the majority of cases, those outdated advertisements are all they can think of. It's quite sad to think that these types of images are so intricately linked to how a newly diagnosed person could determine their outcome. But on the flipside, it's also pretty encouraging to personally know how much things have actually changed in terms of positive disease management and the treatment of MS.

And just as hard as that first consultation can be, so too are the subsequent ones. Everyone processes information at different speeds and there will be patients who need more time to contemplate and then of course, those who leave the initial appointment feeling brave and supported but then jump onto the internet and read far too much – often taking things out of context or using websites that will frighten the heck out them.

In fact, I'll have patients that just unravel after reading information from the wrong sites or social media sources. It's so hard... It's just devastating at times trying to bring them back from hysteria. And again, it's all about the mindset of the patient. Two people can read the same thing and yet have polar opposite reactions. Some will just give up the minute they hear the diagnosis and others find a strength they never knew they had. I'll work with my disheartened patients using examples of the ones who have found that strength and try to convince them that their outlook for their disease course can be very, very good.

Dealing with the diagnosis of a life-altering disease such as MS is such a personalised experience that will obviously differ from person to person. I've got to be able to work out pretty quickly the psyche of a person, what their priorities might be and what type of information or support they'll need most. For some people it's going to be a challenge to process the information, others I'll need to coach out of denial, and others again just take the diagnosis in their stride from the beginning. I've had one instance where I taught the patient how to manage their injectable treatment the day they were diagnosed because they were unquestionably ready for that.

It's these early consultations in particular that you become the carer, the counsellor and the nurse all rolled up into one. Intuition plays a fair factor and the more you deal with people in these situations the better you get at it.

I find it really important to be guided by what our doctors have experienced with the patient as well. This includes everything from understanding a patient history the doctor or neurologist will have gathered, right through to the MRI reports from the radiologists and the neurologist's own interpretation of those. All these elements tell an important story and it's often the doc-tors and the neurologists who are the first to gauge the emotion and disposition of the patient.

I do see a pattern in the types of questions people ask at the varying points of their disease course and it generally correlates to where they're at in life. For young women, I'll initially get the 'will I end up in a wheelchair?' or 'can I still have babies?' questions. Followed by 'will my children get MS?'

After we've discussed those lofty questions about how MS might affect someone's future hopes, then I see people start to recalibrate and think about the 'now.' The patients – and often their families – will start asking what they can do aside from medications to help manage MS. And we now have a great volume of evidence and information about using lifestyle factors to assist in controlling disease progression, so factors such as smoking and exercise and vitamin D can be discussed. And I believe there's plenty of room to incorporate both positive lifestyle changes and natural therapies into the treatment of MS, with the caveat that natural therapies are supervised by a medical team to avoid potential conflicts and side effects with the clinical treatments.

***

I think I take some of my own strength to deal with things from my patients.

I may not have MS but I can certainly empathise with those young people who sit across from me, trying to comprehend the diagnosis; trying to figure out what lies ahead and how it will impact their dreams for the future. My own life has also been filled with those significant life events that we strive towards; love, babies, embarking on a career and then trying to progress through your career so that you can not only make a difference to those you treat but provide your own family with advantages. I've made mistakes along the way and had my own health dilemmas to contend with. So whilst I don't have MS, I understand what it's like for a young woman or man to have the normal pressures of life. I know I have empathy for the way that life doesn't always work out the way you think it will and unfortunate life events rarely happen when you're actually prepared for them.

And the experiences of some of those recent health scares I've faced have been used to reshape my own skills and support for my patients. It's very interesting being on the other side of the desk... One example that really sticks in my mind is how easy it is for people to hear very different things to what's actually been said. And the way that doctors can throw numbers and percentages at you, but they mean very little to a patient in the thick of things. In fact, those figures are likely to confuse you even further during the initial appointments. There's only so much information that will sink in when you're already dealing with a life-changing diagnosis. All-in-all, facing a health scare myself has taught me how to judge people's needs in a different way; it's enabled me to develop a deeper level of empathy.

Over the course of my career, I've seen patients do amazing things after nasty flares and with worsening symptoms. They'll go to rehab, they'll work with the specialists and they'll get their mind around the situation at hand. It all comes down to a determined mindset and what lengths you'll go to get yourself on top of things. They are the people who look at what needs doing and move forward and throw everything they've got at it; they really do work hard at giving themselves the best chance possible. I find that strength of mind and courage amazing.

In its rawest form they just won't allow MS to take control of them. They don't let MS get in the way of their desire to succeed at anything they put their mind to. I've seen people push themselves athletically, undertake massive fundraisers for research, make a career change or conversely, leave their career behind in pursuit of a simpler and more sustainable lifestyle.

They're not letting the disease take charge. They've decided to take full control. I think I take some of my own strength to deal with things from my patients.

I love it when my patients email me and tell me about their triumphs or how they're just getting on with living life. Or they email to tell me about a trip they're going on or a challenge they're undertaking but they'll need advice and help to plan it. It might be accommodating a variation in their meds or managing particular symptoms. I will always have enough time to read those emails and help my patients towards their dreams no matter how much co-ordination is required. It's one of my biggest joys! And we're lucky to have a great network of MS nurses around the world to help facilitate those requests.

Seeing the positive outcomes keeps me going during those more challenging days or throughout the disappointments. And even though sometimes patients choose a different direction to what I would have taken, it's still a satisfying feeling to know I was there to help them process all the information as much as I could and help them in their journey to making that decision. So despite the decision not always going the way I'd like, I feel the patient is better off than if I wasn't there to help and support them with their choices; at least they didn't feel alone in making the decision.

But sadly, there's certainly plenty of people living with MS who do struggle with taking control, particularly after a relapse. Just as defiance can be used for a positive and optimistic outcome against MS, sometimes I see that defiance turn against the patient too; they become defiant – possibly defeated – in a different way. I once had a young patient who I really felt could benefit from using a walking stick. I wanted to prevent any further falls and I knew the walking aid would help conserve energy as well. But this patient was defiant that they wouldn't and couldn't be seen with a stick, no matter the advantages. In the end, the patient decided it was easier to stay at home and it saddened me to see the defiance become a tool that ended up creating an agonising isolation.

I haven't given up on this patient. I truly believe the social aspects of using a stick and being able to get out more will be tremendously beneficial. I have a great relationship with the patient – and they trust me – but we're still not quite at that point of using the stick. And while I see using a stick a big step forward because their quality of life would improve, this person see's the opposite; nearly as if the MS is taking part of them away. Isn't the mind a funny thing?

The type of situations I find challenging are when a patient presents with serious relapses or worsening symptoms and they're already on the best treatment possible for them. It's a situation that doesn't leave a lot of room for movement and I'll admit I can find it hard to know what to do, other than bring the neurologists back in to assess. When you've systematically work through every scenario to problem solve and still can't find a solution, that's when things get frustrating. And this can cover everything from seemingly simple things as injection site reactions through to serious progression of the disease.

And another circumstance I find both challenging and heartbreaking is if a patient has an inher-ent lack of support in managing the disease. Sometimes I wish I could clone myself and go there and help that person but it's just not possible or practical. Generally, these support issues are very tricky to try and sort out as well – particularly when government agencies are involved – because we want it fixed now and we want it fixed without undue cost, but things don't work that way.

And this is where I think sharing insights and experiences can be important. It goes such a long way in being able to offer each other – nurses and patients alike – practical and heartfelt solutions. I especially love hearing from other patients about what works for them and what doesn't. It's great to be able to share those tips amongst everyone. But frustratingly, one of the greatest disservices we contend with now as nurses is social and digital media. If a patient starts trawling through blogs without knowing what's reputable or meaningful or even remotely rational, they can do more damage than good. I'm often having to sort out people after they've read poor (and even dangerous) information. Maybe I need to research all the social media and websites further so I can provide better advice to my patients but it's hard to stay on top of it all.

I think instead some of the best advice I could give to someone newly diagnosed is to empower yourself with well-researched and rational knowledge and to be in contact with the right people and stay on top of your health. Forging those links between your GP, your neurologist and your MS nurse and making sure everyone is communicating effectively and accurately is just so critical. And above all, get to know the condition and your own body and become your own health advocate.

***

Being part of the bigger picture is an important role of the MS nurse.

Maybe it harks back to my fascination with the psychology of social interactions, but I find it quite interesting to work out the various risk profiles of my patient's and how this factors into their decision making process to take a certain type of medication or the chances they're willing to take (or not take) with treatments and any side effects. Once again, there's no firm guide for this; it's so unique to each person's circumstances at that point in time. But that's the primary role of the MS nurse; to discuss the various options, the side effects of medications, the trade-off or potential for disease progression and the effects of that. I think a big part of my interactions with patients is presenting information and advice via a 'risk versus the benefit' approach of anything related to MS.

With the advent of more treatment options also comes the frustration of managing treatment compliance. An oral tablet that should be taken every day is actually not going to be terribly effective if it's only taken three times a week. And compliance from the patient can be tricky as there's so many reasons why they may not adhere to the regimented dose, such as experiencing memory or cognitive decline. Depression in patients can also affect their perspective of what is a priority and what isn't.

And another consideration to be cognizant of is that sometimes the patient will feel far worse whilst taking the disease modifying therapy (DMT) and so yet again, the inclination to comply with their regimen is eroded. And unfortunately, patient anecdotes of how woeful they are made to feel from their DMT are not uncommon. In cases like this, it's my job to teach them the role of their treatment in the greater scheme of things. I handle these situations by being honest and upfront in what to expect, explaining that many of the treatments are designed to delay any disability and prevent relapses and also new lesions from turning up on the MRIs. It's all about providing knowledge and education to the patient and their families.

Treatment non-compliance can be such a big issue, but we have so many little tips to help people out, from just ensuring the meds are in a highly visible place (especially if there's no children in the house) through to setting a recurring alert on the mobile phone as a reminder. Creating a strategy in conjunction with the patient from the beginning helps immensely. And often those strategies are quite simple but I find the key is identifying the type of personality I'm dealing with and figuring out how I can help that person individually.

Matching the DMTs to the person is obviously important for a whole range of reasons. We have to weigh up contra-indications of other health problems that may be existing, we have to look at everything clinically and radiologically and also look at the type of support systems the patient has around them, or conversely, if that support is lacking. First and foremost, the patient is the priority and we have to listen to what they want whilst also ensuring they're making decisions as rationally as possible and with the best information at hand. And if this means that either the clinical team or the patient needs to seek a second opinion, then I'm fully supportive of that.

For someone dealing with poor cognition problems, a daily oral tablet may not be the most suitable choice, instead, coming in for a less frequent treatment such as an infusion of the DMT will provide confirmed compliance. So on top of working with the neurologists to determine the most appropriate treatment for a patient's symptoms and pre-existing conditions, we're also looking further down the track at side effects and the best method of delivery to ensure compliance and taking into account a person's disposition, lifestyle and habits. Yes – we need to be part psychologist, part life coach, part counsellor, part mind readers and I can personally say I have no formal training in any of those things! At times it can be overwhelming, but over the years, experience has provided me with great insights into the techniques that work and those that don't. Regardless, I often think to myself that further formalised training in the psychological aspects of my job would be tremendously beneficial.

I'm fortunate and grateful to work with a great team of specialists in a variety of other areas such as rehabilitation, physiotherapy, social work and neuro-psychology and I've been able to approach them for guidance: Getting advice from colleagues is invaluable. I'm not always the right person to help a patient with particular problems, but I want my patients to know they can come to me with anything so as I can at least guide them towards the right specialist for their needs. Being part of the bigger picture is an important role of the MS nurse and often my role isn't fixing the problem but at least getting them on a path towards a solution. And being a part of the solution is always rewarding to feel.

***

If there's one thing I've learned over the twenty-five years I've been a nurse, it's that I have to make time for me and time for my family and I also make sure I factor in time for exercise and my own well-being. My recent health scare was a good wakeup call as it reinforced my need to prioritise my own health – as much for me as for others. Deleting or eliminating things that aren't important was another big thing I started to embrace. I was very much a 'yes' person. I'd say 'yes' to community activities, 'yes' to my kid's school and 'yes' to pretty much everything. Those little 'yes' activities really built up over time and once I started saying 'no' a little more often, I realised how much I was actually doing that I didn't need to be.

My own health scare forced me to examine everything I was taking on in my life and the positive lesson I took from this situation was I needed to declutter a lot of things that weren't needed. I don't think I would have gone through my decluttering and reprioritisation exercise otherwise, and I'm actually glad I was forced to slow down and rethink. It was the first time I realised I'm not bullet proof and life is too short: I was forced to face my mortality. I think it's definitely something my patients go through at times.

Seeing the positive outcomes is really what keeps me going within my career. And being a MS nurse is such a rewarding calling in general. However, if I had a genie come out of a bottle and provide me unlimited resources, I'd simply ask for more help. I know two of us could do this job far better than one. Imagine if I could spend more time with my patients or just spend time with each and every patient registered at our clinic? We have hundreds of patients in our MS clinic at St Vincent's and I can't physically or logistically see everyone. And they might not need my help anyway, but wouldn't it be great for the patients to feel reassured that they always had that resource?

My hopes for the future treatment and management of MS:

•   There will definitely be a cure in our lifetime. Only twenty years ago it was the norm to depict people with MS as being in wheelchairs. Fast forward to today and we know so much more about the disease and we have more effective drugs, and a greater range of DMTs available to treat MS. Some of these DMTs are so effective that we're seeing a reduction of lesions and relapses by up to 80 percent. Surely a cure is the next milestone? I'd rather be out of a job any day if it meant we could find a cure.

•   Do you want to know how I know we're advancing in unravelling the mysteries of MS? It's because I find it hard to keep up with the volume of information and research about the cause, the cure and disease management. It's a good problem to have – to have to stay on top of so many positive developments and new insights. I just want my patients to have as many options as possible.

My advice for nurses beginning their career:

•   Get to know your MS nursing colleagues. Initially I came into this specialist field not having any clue at all. Building a solid network or people around me has been essential – from the neurologists, allied health care team, to the other MS nurses around the country and right through to the other specialists in therapy, psychology and psychiatry. As important as it is for a patient to have their own support network, it's important for us nurses to have a similar resource.

•   I believe the dynamic of teamwork is one of the most enjoyable experiences of this job and it's important to both seek advice and offer input so as you can create the best outcome for the patient and also just have a rewarding career experience.

BIOGRAPHIES

Kaye D Hooper, RN RM BA MPH
Royal Brisbane and Women's Hospital, Australia

Kaye first started work in the world of MS in 1994 as a MS research nurse with Professor Michael Pender based at University of Queensland in Brisbane. In 1996 she took on the role of Manager and MS Clinical Nurse Consultant at the newly established MS Clinic, Royal Brisbane and Women's Hospital / University of Queensland.

During the past 25 years Kaye has worked in MS research, MS clinical patient care and support, patient and family education and provided MS education and support for other nurses and health professionals. Kaye is a founding Board member of IOMSN (International Organization of MS Nurses) and founding President of MSNA (MS Nurses Australasia); she has served on Boards of different MS organisations; authored and co-authored articles and booklets for journals and MS organisations; and been an invited speaker at national and international MS meetings.

Kaye is inspired by her patients as they live courageously with the ups and downs of MS and she treasures the friendships she has made with MS colleagues around the world who have shared the journey with her over these past 25 years.

June Halper, MSN, APN-C, MSCN, FAAN
Consortium of Multiple Sclerosis Centers, USA

June Halper is a certified adult nurse practitioner who has specialised in multiple sclerosis since 1978. She is the Chief Executive Officer of the Consortium of Multiple Sclerosis Centers (CMSC) and Executive Director of the IOMSN.

Ms. Halper has published and lectured extensively on multiple sclerosis and its ramifications. Her numerous publications include Comprehensive Nursing Care in Multiple Sclerosis and Advanced Concepts in Nursing Care in Multiple Sclerosis, co-editor of Staying Well with Multiple Sclerosis: A Self-Care Guide, and co-editor of Nursing Practices in Multiple Sclerosis: A Core Curriculum. She is a member of the American Academy of Nurse Practitioners, the founding director of IOMSN, the International Organization of MS Nurses, and the recipient of the IOMSN's first June Halper Award for Excellence in Nursing in Multiple Sclerosis. She was inducted as a Fellow into the American Academy of Nursing in November 1999. In 2000, she spearheaded the establishment of the Multiple Sclerosis International Certification Board who developed the first international certification examination in multiple sclerosis nursing offered in June 2002 and bi-annually thereafter. As CEO of the CMSC, she initiated the first certification examination for MS specialists in 2004.

As early as 1995, Ms. Halper was involved in the development of clinical practice guidelines in multiple sclerosis which were multi-organization collaborative projects. She was involved in the publication of guidelines in bladder dysfunction in MS, fatigue in MS, spasticity in MS, immunizations in MS, and disease modification in MS. Subsequently the CMSC has adopted a best practices model and Ms. Halper was involved in publication of models of comprehensive care, complex symptomatic management, and cognition to name a few publications. (please visit www.mscare.org for a full listing)

In 1995 the NARCOMS patient registry was established under Ms. Halper's leadership and support. Since that time the registry has been a source of information about outcome measures and a resource for quality improvement projects.

***

Joelle Massouh, BSN, RN
AUBMC Multiple Sclerosis Center, Beirut, Lebanon

Ms. Massouh is the Nurse in Charge at the Nehme and Therese Tohme Multiple Sclerosis Center, American University of Beirut Medical Center (AUBMC), in Beirut, Lebanon. She received her Bachelor of Science in Nursing from the American University of Beirut in 2007 along with a minor in Psychology.

She is the first nurse and healthcare professional in the Middle East to be double certified as a Multiple Sclerosis Certified Nurse (MSCN) by the Multiple Sclerosis Nursing International Certification Board (MSNICB), and as a Multiple Sclerosis Certified Specialist (MSCS) by the Consortium of Multiple Sclerosis Centers (CMSC). She is a member of the International Organization of Multiple Sclerosis Nurses (IOMSN) and a board member representing the Middle East on the MSNICB.

Ms. Massouh is also the Nursing Program Coordinator of the Middle East North Africa Committee for Treatment and Research in MS (MENACTRIMS); she organizes the full day parallel nursing session at the annual MENACTRIMS congress and passionately advocates for advancing the specialty of MS nursing in the MENA region.

In 2019, she was awarded the inaugural International MS Nursing Leadership Award by IOMSN at the annual CMSC congress in USA.

***

Astrid Slettenaar, RN, MSCN, MANP
Medisch Spectrum Twente, Netherlands

Astrid Slettenaar is a nurse practitioner at the MS Center at Medisch Spectrum Twente; a general hospital in the east of the Netherlands. She joined the department in 1996 and assumed her nurse practitioner position in 2009. Astrid is also the president of the Dutch Foundation of Masters in MS. As an active member she participated in several projects to create a higher quality in the care for people with MS. The board members of the Foundation developed the "Dutch Guideline Adherence to the First-line Injection Therapy in Multiple Sclerosis" in 2015. The guideline describes the factors that influence adherence, such as flu-like symptoms injection site reactions, fatigue, depression, anxiety and cognitive dysfunction.

Astrid wrote a cookbook for patients with MS, called 'Delicious Meals Made Simple,' that has found its way to patients in several countries in four languages. She was one of the developers the Multiple Shaker App and teachers nursing students research and MS. She started her second term as a board member of the Multiple Sclerosis International Certification Board.

Jennifer R. Boyd, RN, BScN, MHSc, CNN(C), MSCN
The Hospital for Sick Children, Toronto, Ontario, Canada

Jennifer Boyd has been a Clinical Nurse Specialist in Neurology since 1996. In addition to her broad nursing expertise in child neurology, she has subspecialty interest and advanced knowledge in the care of patients with neuromuscular disorders, infantile spasms, new onset seizures and multiple sclerosis (MS). She is recognized internationally as an expert in the nursing care of children and adolescents with MS. Jennifer obtained her Bachelor of Science in Nursing from the University of Western Ontario and Master of Health Sciences from McMaster University. She has her Certification in Neuroscience Nursing in Canada – CNN(C), and is a Multiple Sclerosis Certified Nurse – MSCN. She is also an Adjunct Lecturer with the Lawrence S. Bloomberg Faculty of Nursing at the University of Toronto and a Project Investigator with the SickKids Research Institute. Active in numerous professional organizations, Jennifer is a Past President of the Association of Child Neurology Nurses (2009-2011), a former member of the Board of Directors of the International Organization of Multiple Sclerosis Nurses (2006-2012) and is currently a member of the Multiple Sclerosis Nurses International Certification Board (2016-). Jennifer is a peer-reviewer for manuscripts submitted to the Canadian Journal of Neuroscience Nursing, and frequently writes and presents on topics relating to child neurology nursing.

***

Dr. Therese Burke, RN, MSCN, PhD.
University of Notre Dame University, Sydney, Australia

Therese Burke has been a MS Nurse in Australia for over 15 years, working in both clinical and research nursing roles, and is currently a post-doctoral researcher in the School of Nursing at The University of Notre Dame in Sydney. Therese completed her PhD in

February 2019, using qualitative inquiry to explore the life trajectory of people living with Relapsing Remitting Multiple Sclerosis. Several international publications have resulted from this research, including the British Journal of Neuroscience Nursing, Research Theory and Practice and the Australian Journal of Advanced Nursing. Therese is a Past President of MS Nurses Australasia and has also been a member of the IOMSN MS Nurses International Certification Board since 2011, currently serving as the Immediate Past President and Recertification Chair.

Therese was presented the John Studdy award from MS Australia in 2016 for her contribution to MS research and clinical care in Australia, and also the June Halper award from IOMSN for contributions to international MS care in the same year.

Current post-doctoral research interests include the transition from RRMS to SPMS from the patient perspective, the effects of a diagnosis of CIS on patients and MS nurses and exploring the role definition and education needs of MS Nurses.

***

Megan Weigel, DNP, ARNP-C, APHN-C, MSCN
First Coast Integrative Medicine, USA

Megan Weigel, DNP, is a nurse practitioner specializing in neurological care in Jacksonville Beach, FL, where she brings a unique integrative medicine and holistic nursing perspective to her practice, First Coast Integrative Medicine. She has been a Multiple Sclerosis certified nurse since 2005, and an NP for 18 years. She is also a board certified Advanced Practice Holistic Nurse.

She earned her doctorate of nursing practice from the University of Florida, where her research emphasis was on preventive health-care. She was recognized as one of Jacksonville Business Journal's "40 Under 40" and as an Outstanding Young Alumnus of the University of Florida in 2010, and as one of the "Great 100 Nurses of Northeast Florida" in 2015. She completed a fellowship in Integrative Medicine at the University of Arizona in the Fall of 2018, which complements her practice focus on wellness and holistic care.

She is the past-president of the International Organization of MS Nurses, serves on the editorial board of the International Journal of MS Care, and enjoyed years of service on the Healthcare Advisory Committee for her local National MS Society chapter. She is the co-founder of oMS Yoga, a non-profit organization that brings free yoga classes to people living with MS along the east coast. She is a yogi, surfer, runner, avid reader, writer, and enjoys her work in the neurology field immensely, especially educating people living with neurological issues and peers about the importance of wellness as an integral part of treatment. She is an invited speaker nationally on these subjects. Megan is a wife and mother who understands the importance of one's personal story, the search for meaning and the value of relationships.

***

Michael Mortensen, RN, MS specialist nurse
MS Limited (formerly MS Society of Tasmania), Australia

Michael Mortensen has spent the last ten years as a MS Specialist Nurse and also assisted as the backup study coordinator on several clinical trials at Royal Hobart Hospital. Additionally, Michael has participated in a number of pharmaceutical advisory boards. His current focus is assisting clients to gain access to the National Disability Insurance Scheme in Australia.

Del Thomas, RN, MSCN
Wye Valley NHS Trust, United Kingdom

Del Thomas is an MS Clinical Nurse Specialist working in Herefordshire for the Wye Valley NHS Trust. Del has been an MS Nurse for over 12 years and is Co-Chair of the UK MS Specialist Nurse Association and a board member of the International Organization of MS Nurses (IOMSN). Del is also a Clinical Editor on MS publication MS Today.

In 2016, Del was named the Outstanding MS Specialist Nurse in the QuDos in MS Awards. She has also published two significant research papers, 'The Evolving Role of the Multiple Sclerosis Nurse – Implications of Future Management Directions' and 'The International Multiple Sclerosis Clinic – A Virtual Tour of Best Practice Multiple Sclerosis Nursing.'

***

Susan Agland, MNurs (Research), RN, MSCN
John Hunter Hospital, Australia

Susan Agland is a clinical nurse specialist in Multiple Sclerosis at the John Hunter Hospital in Newcastle, NSW. Susan was first lured into the world of MS through the Ausimmune study, collecting data on various environmental factors associated with MS. Since its launch in 2006 Susan has been part of the multidisciplinary clinic providing care to people with MS in the Hunter New England Region and beyond. During this time Susan has added to her post basic qualification; a Masters in Nursing Research, examining the role of stress management in MS. She is a strong advocate for the MS Nurse Specialist role in improving health outcomes and minimising the impact of neurological disease on the lives of people with MS.

In Memoriam
Nicola 'Nicki' Ward-Abel

Nicki Ward-Abel was involved in the world of MS for over 20 years and was one of the first MS nurses in the United Kingdom. In her later career, she was a Lecturer Practitioner in MS at Birmingham City University and worked as a MS nurse at the Queen Elizabeth Hospital in Birmingham.

Education was her underlying mantra, and she strove to create and impart resources for her fellow nurses and patients alike. She was recognised for developing a fatigue management program for patients and one of her specialty interest areas was sexual dysfunction; when you heard one of Nicki's talks about sexual dysfunction, you certainly didn't forget it in a hurry! No subject was off-limits.

However it was her contribution to MS nurse education through which she made the biggest impact, both within the UK and internationally. She was known for her driving passion to set MS nurses apart in terms of their knowledge-base. She was instrumental in developing the degree module for new MS nurses going through university in the UK and would always go the extra mile to support and nurture the next generation of MS nurses.

She was one of the founding committee members of the UKMSSNA, again striving to improve accessibility to knowledge and education for MS nurses. She was also instrumental in establishing the Multiple Sclerosis International Certification Board and enjoyed working with the International Organization of MS Nurses. She had also been involved in the compilation of MS Nurse-Pro, the European online MS nurse's education program.

Nicki sadly passed away in September 2018 after a courageous battle with cancer. I feel truly blessed that I was able to interview her for this book in April of that year. She was an inspiration to all who knew her, always showing courage and determination to not give in, and she has left a gaping hole in the life of everyone who knew her.

***

Karen Vernon, RGN, BSc (Hons), Post Grad Dip, MSCN, NMP Manchester Centre of Clinical Neuroscinces (MSCCN) MS Service, United Kingdom

Karen Vernon is the Nurse Consultant in Multiple Sclerosis of the MS Service which is based MSCCN, Salford Royal NHS Foundation Trust, one of the leading MS Centres in the UK. Karen is one of three people in the county who, currently, hold the title of MS Nurse Consultant.

Karen has worked in neurology for longer than she cares to remember! From being a ward manager on an acute neurology ward, to becoming a community neurology nurse to specialising in MS at different centres, to where Karen is today. She has helped to recruit patients to clinical trials both for MS and Parkinsons disease and was part of the steering group that devised a clinical audit tool for MS nurses which is now used across the UK.

Aside from the advances for patients, Karen considers one of the overwhelming positives in MS care has been the development of the MS specialist nurse role and it is the future proofing of the role that she is passionate about. The equity of service provision to patients with MS is currently another priority for her.

Karen was co-chair of the United Kingdom Multiple Sclerosis Specialist Nurse Association (UKMSSNA) and is currently the

UK representative on the Multiple Sclerosis Nurses International Certification Board (MSNICB).

She has been involved in MS research projects with both Salford and Nottingham University, looking at varying aspects of MS care. Karen has co-authored a number of MS publications over the years and has also had the opportunity to make platform presentations at national and international MS conferences in addition to having numerous poster presentations accepted.

Along with 2 of her Consultant colleagues, Karen has developed an award-winning neurological examination course for MS nurses to help them enhance their skills.

***

Edith Cinc, RN
N-CRESS, Austin Health, Victoria, Australia

Edith Cinc is an MS Research & Immunotherapy Support Nurse at N-CRESS - the Neuro-Immunology Clinical Research, Education and Support Service at Austin Health in Victoria, Australia. Edith draws on an extensive background in oncology and haematology to now specialise in managing MS patients transitioning to immunosuppressant and biological therapies. She utilises a multidisciplinary approach to develop patient management tools and protocols specifically targeted to this patient population. Edith's role and professional interests include counselling and education spanning both research and clinical domains. Her goal for all people with MS is to be well informed to empower themselves to optimise self care and management of their disease.

Anne Krakau Hansen, RN, MSCN
Danish Multiple Sclerosis Center, Rigshospitalet Copenhagen, Denmark

Anne Krakau is the head Nurse in the Danish Multiple Sclerosis Center, Rigshospitalet Copenhagen.

She became a nurse in 1983. Worked in the first years in the medical, rheumatological, physiurgical and psychiatric field. Since 1990, she has been a neurological nurse and has gained her specialist education in this specialty. In 1996, she started working with special care and treatment for multiple sclerosis patients. Since January 2000 she has been employed by the Danish Multiple Sclerosis Center, Rigshospitalet Copenhagen. Since 2006 as leading (head) nurse. There are 15 nurses employed exclusively to treat MS patients in the out-patient clinic. Associated with approximately 3800 patients.

Anne is the chairman of the Danish MS Nurses association.

***

Adriana Cartwright, RN, MSCN
St Vincent's Hospital, Melbourne, Australia

Adriana Cartwright completed her Bachelor of Nursing and commenced working at St Vincent's as a Registered Nurse 1994 and has since remained mostly in the area of Neurosurgery. During her time in Acute Care, she worked in various roles such as Clinical Nurse Specialist and as an Associate Nurse Unit Manager. During this time, Adriana also completed a Diploma of Frontline Management and a Post Graduate Certificate in Neurosciences Nursing. In 2008, she commenced in the role of Clinical Nurse Educator for the post-graduate Neurosciences Nursing course.

In 2010 she commenced in her role as a Stroke Research Coordinator and the next year as the MS Nurse and MS Clinical Trial Coordinator in the Neuro Immunology Unit. In 2013, Adriana undertook (and has since maintained) her Multiple Sclerosis Certified Nurse (MSCN) qualification with the Multiple Sclerosis Nurses International Certification Board (MSNICB).

Adriana continues to work in a multi-disciplinary team at the Department of Clinical Neurosciences and Neurological Research at St Vincent's hospital in Melbourne, where she works alongside a dedicated team of neurologists to provide a complete clinical and diagnostic service and is also actively involved in clinical trials and research projects.

ACKNOWLEDGEMENTS

Across the course of my journalism career, I'm certain I've written more words than what's contained in all three books in the Taking Control series, yet writing these books has been one of the most challenging (and exhilarating) things I've ever done.

You see, life goes on around you when you write a book. I wish I could tell you I closeted myself away in a seaside villa in the south of France whilst I tapped away on an antique typewriter every day, only pausing to replenish my alternating mugs of coffee or Scotch whiskey.... but I didn't. (Hmmmm... maybe next time...) Other projects came and went. Some incredibly time-consuming and exceptionally worthy and yet others quite mundane but utterly necessary. And in amongst all that, I was managing the daily fluctuation of MS symptoms, which frankly, were quite annoying and often frustratingly debilitating.

But I always had immense inspiration and support at hand and this never ceased to keep me driven and focused.

First and foremost I want to acknowledge my family. Mum, Dad and Rachel.... you kept me level and built my confidence when it was down and you never stopped reminding me why I was doing this. You supported in me in more ways than people will ever know to bring this series to life. Any appreciation for this book series is yours to be shared.

Mon ami, Louise... my tour manager. The inspiration behind every 'pens down' celebration and the instigator to taking this project global.... with any excuse what-so-ever! Your friendship, support and rationality is one of the best things in my life and you keep me sane when I write.

Most importantly, to the MS nurses I interviewed for this book. Kaye, Therese, Megan, Joelle, June, Jennifer, Susan, Michael, Astrid, Del, Karen, Angel Nicki, Edith, Adriana and Anne. Thankyou for opening your lives to me and trusting me with your thoughts and fears and hopes and insights. It takes a lot to bare your soul and you did so in good faith that it would help others. That is the true spirit of compassion. Your stories are remarkable. There were times in crafting the chapters that I would literally sit at my laptop and sob. And other times I'd sit there giggling because I could hear your voice in the jokes and sage advice as I typed the words. You have all changed me irrevocably and undoubtedly made me stronger. You are simply the best.

***

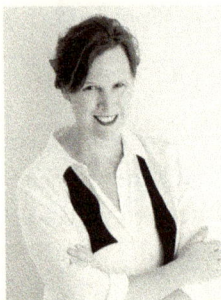

ABOUT THE AUTHOR

Jillian is an award-winning journalist who concentrated primarily on business and motoring writing before turning her hand to authoring books in 2012 when she was diagnosed with Multiple Sclerosis at the age of 42. Taking Control Compassionately is Jillian's fourth book.

Community and philanthropy are ingrained into Jillian's spirit and she works with numerous organisations to raise awareness and funds for health and medical research in areas close to her heart.

She is immensely proud to be an ambassador for global initiative Kiss Goodbye to MS and also spent two years as the writer in residence for MS Research Australia. Both of these roles have afforded tremendous opportunities, such as speaking at Australia's Parliament House on World MS Day in 2018 and being invited onto the foundation team of 'Stop and Reverse MS' – a global strategic initiative to drastically reduce the time it will take to find a cure for MS from 40 years down to just 10 years via accelerated medical research.

All of these experiences have fuelled Jillian's primary passion; to drive systemic change through story telling. In her 'spare' time, she has also written two best-selling books and worked as a ghost-writer. Jillian travels extensively – a great perk of being a speaker and a writer – and something she engineered soon after her diagnosis with MS so she could live life to the fullest.